TRIAGE AND JUSTICE

TRIAGE AND JUSTICE

Gerald R. Winslow

UNIVERSITY OF CALIFORNIA PRESS
Berkeley   Los Angeles   London

University of California Press
Berkeley and Los Angeles, California

University of California Press, Ltd.
London, England

Library of Congress Cataloging in Publication Data
Winslow, Gerald R.
    Triage and justice.

    Bibliography
    Includes index.
    1. Triage (Medicine)—Moral and religious
aspects. 2. Social justice. I. Title.
R725.5.W56   174' .2   81–10434
ISBN 0–520–04328–6   AACR2

Printed in the United States of America

1 2 3 4 5 6 7 8 9

To Betty Jean

Contents

vii

Contents

Preface

The need to ration life-saving resources presents modern medicine with one of its most difficult moral issues. Both medical needs and the human ability to produce new and often costly therapies are virtually unlimited. Thus, there is an emerging awareness that not all medical treatments can be made available to everyone in need, even when life is at stake. Some method of coping with scarcities inevitably develops. And with it comes the debate about the morality of rationing, or *triage*, as it has become known.

It is my purpose in this work to consider alternative approaches to triage in the light of a theory of social justice. As I understand them, questions of social justice are, to a large extent, questions about the distribution of burdens and benefits within the context of social institutions. The health care system, as it has developed in this century, is unquestionably a social institution of great importance. The time is past when the most significant questions of health care distribution had to do with the way individual practitioners apportioned their time and services. Modern medicine is a complicated network of social roles and practices, complex financial arrangements, and a system of rules, both written and unwritten, which specify permissible activities and establish sanctions for misconduct. Moreover, as social institutions go, the present health care system distributes many benefits held in unusually high esteem and burdens increasingly perceived as unbearable. Such a social institution invites scrutiny of its distributional patterns from the perspective of justice. This is especially true in the case of triage when the benefits in question are both scarce and life-saving.

In order to facilitate an evaluation of various approaches to triage, I make use of John Rawls's social-contract theory of justice. The decision to discuss triage in terms of Rawls's theory may need little defense. Perhaps it is enough to recognize that a significant problem of justice is being examined in the light of one of the most important treatments of social justice in modern times. But there are more specific reasons for the choice. Rawls's work takes up explicitly the problems of utility, efficiency, and equality which have also been at the center of concern over triage. What is more, Rawls's theory represents an ambitious and creative attempt to rank principles of justice. Thus, I will argue, the theory provides a useful framework within which approaches to triage can be rejected, selected, and ordered. In turn, the problems of triage may show us aspects of Rawls's theory needing modification.

The chief result of this examination of triage is an argument for the limitation of utilitarian considerations and for the establishment of a basic presumption in favor of providing equal access to the scarce medical resources for those who are in need. I cannot claim, of course, to be the first to offer such an argument. But I have attempted to provide a more thorough discussion of the options and a more complete system for evaluating them.

It is my hope that this work will be of interest to those who study ethics, especially biomedical ethics. But I have tried to produce a discussion that will attract readers engaged in health care provision and planning, as well as those who ''do ethics.'' The risks of such boundary crossing are quite obvious. But I am convinced that the issues of triage merit the attempt.

I wish that my gratitude to those who have helped me with this project could be distributed fairly. But the work has continued a long time, and my debts are many. I must mention only a special few. My thanks go first to Karen Lebacqz, my advisor throughout my studies at the Graduate Theological Union and the coordinator of the dissertation committee that read the original version of this work. Lebacqz has given steady encouragement, keen scholarly insights, and sincere personal concern. I also owe large debts of gratitude to Albert Jonsen of the University of California, San Francisco; Thomas Schubeck of the Graduate Theological Union; and Professor Roy Branson of the Kennedy Institute for Bioethics. They each offered extensive suggestions and criticisms. My initial conversations about triage were with Bruce MacIntyre of Carroll College while he was on sabbatical leave in Berkeley. Those discussions have continued to have an impact on the preparation of this book. Also of special value to me was the time I spent with the Health Policy Program at the University of California, San Francisco. I am grateful to the director of the program, Philip Lee, and to the staff members and fellows who contributed to my understanding of many of the issues related to the topic of this work. None whom I have just named is responsible for the mistakes that remain in my work.

It is also a pleasure to acknowledge the help of my friends at Walla Walla College. The college has supported this project financially and in many other ways. My colleagues in the School of Theology have borne extra burdens so that I could be free to complete this work. One staff member, Ruth Popplewell, has provided outstanding technical assistance in typing and final preparation of the manuscript. And particularly important to me were frequent conversations with my friend and colleague, the late Ruth Burgeson.

Words fall short as I wish to express my deepest appreciation to those whose personal investment has been the greatest. My wife, Betty, has lived with many inconveniences while this work proceeded. During this time, she has offered constant interest and support. When the work became tedious, my daughters, Lisa and Angela, volunteered welcome moments of diversion. I continue to learn the most practical lessons of justice and love from them.

Gerald R. Winslow

Walla Walla College
February 1981

I The Concept of Triage in Modern Medicine

DICTONARY DEFINITIONS SOMETIMES HIDE complexity. Take, for example, one medical dictionary's definition of triage:

> Triage . . . The medical screening of patients to determine their priority for treatment; the separation of a large number of casualties, in military or civilian disaster medical care, into three groups: those who cannot be expected to survive even with treatment, those who will recover without treatment, and the priority group of those who need treatment in order to survive.[1]

By the standards of dictionary definitions, this probably would be judged a good one. It is clear and concise. The three-way division of casualties, for example, seems sensible and easy to understand.

The curious person, however, may be left with some questions. How did a French word which once referred to the grading of agricultural products[2] come to designate the sorting of people needing medical care? What factors seem to have necessitated such triage decisions? And on what grounds have the decisions been made? One cannot expect to find answers to such questions in a dictionary. Behind the neat and orderly definition is the complex tale of an idea.

Triage in Military Medicine

The earliest roots of rational systems of triage are found in military medicine's practice of classifying casualties. Initiation of this procedure has been attributed to Baron Dominique Jean Larrey, Napoleon's chief medical officer.[3] Larrey devoted

1

nearly his entire adult life to military medicine and participated in hundreds of military engagements. By his own account, he once amputated 200 limbs in one twenty-four-hour period.[4] His scrupulous concern for detail and efficiency gave impetus to the development of a number of medical innovations of lasting significance.

One of Larrey's goals was to perform surgery as soon after the injury as possible. For Larrey, this meant taking the medical services into the field and the development of "ambulances," a term that in Larrey's time referred not only to vehicles for transporting the wounded but also to a unit of medical personnel.[5]

Although there seems to be no record of Larrey using the term *triage*, it is clear that his work led in the direction of a "scientific" approach to military medicine, including the sorting of casualties. In his report of the Russian campaign he wrote:

> I had scarcely made the necessary preparations, when the wounded arrived in a crowd, and much confusion would have ensued, had I not pursued the order of dressing and arrangement, observed by me in all battles . . . [6]

Larrey was more than a little proud of the successes of his medical personnel in the field in spite of the scarcity of resources about which he sometimes complained. His explanation of the favorable results is of interest: "This success, if the scarcity of resources . . . be considered is essentially owing to the prompt and methodical succour received by the wounded on the field of battle . . . [7]

An important part of Larrey's "methodical succour" was his principle of sorting casualties on the basis of medical need. In Larrey's words:"[T]hose who are dangerously wounded must be tended first, *entirely without regard to rank or distinction.* Those less severely injured must wait until the gravely wounded have been operated on and dressed."[8] Whether or not this principle was always carried out in practice is probably impossible to determine. What is noteworthy, however, is Larrey's expressed unwillingness to consider factors other than relative levels of medical need. As Stuart Hinds, British physician and medical historian, has noted, " . . . Larrey rejected out of hand any idea of treating persons by priorities other than medical need."[9]

Larrey's work gradually became a model for military medicine throughout the Western world. But the development was slow. In the American Civil War, for example, the ability to treat casualties lagged far behind the destructive capacity of new armaments. Weaponry such as Requa's machine gun, land mines, explosive bullets, and telescopic sights led to enormously high numbers of casualties. But the medical services were so poorly organized, lacking efficient ambulance service, staff, and supplies, that care of the wounded was often haphazard at best.[10]

Literary figure Walt Whitman, who spent much of his time during the Civil War caring for the North's wounded, described the scene. Hundreds of men, he wrote, "bleed to death, or die from exhaustion, either actually untouched at all, or with merely the laying of them down and leaving them, when there ought to be means provided to save them."[11] He went on to protest that there was "no system, no foresight, no genius." Elsewhere he tells of the order in which the wounded were treated. "The men, whatever their condition, lie there, and patiently wait till their turn comes to be taken up."[12] No rationale is offered for this system, or nonsystem, of treating a casualty on the basis of his place in the queue. Perhaps there was none. It seems likely that a beleaguered medical service was simply coping with the situation in the way that seemed best at the time.

Other literature of this period reveals a diversity of precepts concerning the sorting of casualties. One author suggested that all patients be classified "according to the site and nature of their wounds," and then advocated that all cases of a similar nature be brought near one another.[13] Even though little is said about priorities in treatment, presumably this system was thought to be the most efficient. But another writer argued that similar cases should be kept separate in order to prevent the casualties from becoming unduly alarmed about their conditions.[14]

In the case of any of these early systems of casualty sorting, one may wonder how much benefit there was in being given priority when the quality of medical care is considered. The kinds of medical treatments that were being advocated at the time lead one to conclude that the probability of being harmed must have been about as great as that of being helped. For example, the author just cited reassured his fellow medical personnel that ordinarily it would not be necessary to bleed casualties, but, he said, sawdust should be used in every wound to keep maggots from developing.[15]

In the early discussions of casualty sorting, a number of features differ markedly from the triage schemes that developed later. For example, any mention of military usefulness as a criterion for setting priorities seems entirely lacking. Larrey apparently rejected such a standard. Others do not even allude to it. Similarly, no reference is made to the idea that the treatment of some casualties might be too time-consuming, thus hindering the treatment of others or the prosecution of the military effort. It is even difficult, though not impossible, to find mention made of a "hopeless" category of casualties.[16] Given the nature of many of the wounds and the state of the medical art, it seems quite certain that many unsalvageable cases were encountered. But references to such casualties are usually oblique and do not loom large in the discussions of the day. All three of these factors, military usefulness, the availability of time, and the degree of hopelessness take on greater significance in the more sophisticated triage proposals of the twentieth century.

The trench warfare of World War I resulted in an unprecedented number of casualties and with them an unprecedented need for triage. Nearly 8,000,000 men were killed and over 19,000,000 were wounded—nearly twice as many as in World War II.[17] New arsenals, well suited to a war of attrition, included not only many new mechanized weapons and "improved" machine guns, but also phosgene, chlorine, and mustard, an array of deadly gases.

Along with this increased ability to kill and maim, armies were developing new techniques for saving the wounded. One of the most notable of these was the motorized ambulance.[18] This and other changes in the transportation and care of the wounded often resulted in the arrival of enormous numbers of casualties at the "casualty clearing stations" (CCS). In times of heavy fighting it was not uncommon to process between 1000 and 2000 wounded patients in a day. Moreover, the kinds of casualties arriving at a CCS differed from those of earlier times. Rapid transportation and better first-aid techniques made it possible to bring soldiers to the CCS who were so seriously wounded that they almost certainly would have died in the field in earlier times.

Faced with such adverse conditions, the medical personnel at the CCS struggled to find ways to conserve the scarce resources, the most important of which were often their own time and energy. A passage from a medical handbook of that period describes the problem and advocates a response:

[A] hospital with 300 or 400 beds may suddenly be overwhelmed by 1000 or more cases. It is often, therefore, physically impossible to give speedy and thorough treatment to all. A single case, even if it urgently requires attention,—if this will absorb a long time,—may have to wait, for in that same time a dozen others, almost equally exigent, but requiring less time, might be cared for. *The greatest good of the greatest number must be the rule.*[19]

Based on the utilitarian principle—the greatest good of the greatest number—new and sometimes elaborate systems of casualty sorting evolved. The process now came to be referred to as *triage*.[20] Military medical manuals contained not only detailed outlines of triage categories but also diagrams illustrating the location and function of the "Poste de Triage."[21] One searches in vain, however, for the tidy categories that later came to be associated with triage decision making and that are included in the dictionary definition at the beginning of this chapter.

The following summaries of differing triage categories are illustrative of the schemes proposed or in use at the time:

Plan A[22]
1. Those who are severely wounded and cannot be transported
2. Those who are less severely wounded and can be transported
3. Those who are still capable of walking

Plan B[23]
1. Those who can be immediately evacuated
2. Those requiring minor operations
3. Those requiring immediate major operations
4. Those requiring immediate resuscitation

In both of the above schemes there is an attempt to balance a number of factors. Of these, the two most important are the relative urgency of the medical needs and the feasibility of transportation. One can only begin to glimpse the complexity of the factors that had to be included in the calculations if efficiency were to be maintained.

As with earlier schemes of sorting, no mention is made of the hopelessly wounded. Nevertheless, it is certain that such casualties were brought to the CCS's. Laffin confirms this fact in a description of the treatment of casualties during the Battle of Verdun: "The surgeon would indicate that a particular case was rejected and the orderlies would carry him from the operating cellar and put him in the open cover. . . . These men died where they lay."[24]

As seen above, the greatest good of the greatest number was the expressed goal of triage. But during World War I, it became more and more obvious that this utilitarian principle was capable of at least two distinct interpretations when applied to military medicine. First, it was taken to mean saving the lives and limbs of as many casualties as possible. Surgeons were encouraged to avoid the badly wounded in order to work for the "greatest net profit."[25]

Second, another interpretation of the utilitarian principle called for the preservation of military manpower or the maximization of fighting strength. During World War I, there was an increasing emphasis on giving priority to the slightly wounded in order to return them quickly to the battle.[26] In some instances, this rationale predominated. For example, one handbook claimed that the objectives of triage "are twofold: 1st, conservation of manpower; 2nd, the conservation of the interests of the sick and wounded."[27] Even the transportation of ammunition and supplies was sometimes deemed more important than caring for the wounded.[28]

During World War II the basic patterns for triage decision making were further refined.[29] But now one's place in the order of treatment unquestionably made more difference than in the past. Table 1 shows the percentages of American casualties who died of their wounds and gives evidence of the effects of improved medical care in three different wars.[30]

TABLE 1

Percentage of American Casualties Dying of Wounds

War	Years	Number wounded	Percentage of casualties dying of wounds
American Civil War (Union Army)	1861–1865	318,200	14.1
World War I	1917–1918	153,000	8.1
World War II	1941–1945	598,000	4.5

Numerous factors contributed to this decline in the percentages of deaths. Sanitation was better. Transportation was faster. Moreover, a number of new life-saving remedies became available. Most important among these were the antibiotics, sulfa and penicillin, and blood plasma. In contrast with bleeding casualties and putting sawdust in the wound, blood transfusions and the use of sulfa directly in the wounds greatly enhanced the probability of a casualty's survival. At the same time, shortages of such life-saving resources or of the personnel or time to administer them gave an added sense of tragedy to the deaths that thereby ensued. The lack of penicillin during much of World War II was, perhaps, the most dramatic example.

According to Keefer, in the summer of 1941 there was not enough penicillin in the United States to treat a single person.[31] By the spring of 1942 enough of the drug was available to treat *one* patient, and by the summer of that year there was a sufficient amount for about ten patients. From the beginning, excruciating decisions had to be made about the drug's distribution. Investigators were permitted to test the drug in cases that, in Keefer's words, "would yield the maximum information of value to the armed services."[32] It is interesting to note that in this developmental period no patient or doctor was allowed to purchase penicillin, nor was any patient charged for it.

Very early in the testing of penicillin it was discovered that

7

the drug was not only amazingly successful in fighting infections in wounds, but also was the best available treatment for venereal diseases. This fact led to some of the most widely discussed triage decisions of the war. One such well-known story has been recounted by Beecher.[33] Commanders of the American forces in North Africa had to decide whether to use the limited supply of penicillin for battle casualties or for gonorrhea victims. The decision was made to treat those suffering from venereal disease rather than those wounded in battle. To the people in charge, it seemed more reasonable to return to battle readiness those who could be most easily rehabilitated.

This story was not particularly unusual during the war. Hinds tells of a similar case of "penicillin triage" that took place in Great Britain in 1944.[34] The decision was made to give priority in the use of the precious supplies of penicillin to the trainees in the bombing crews who contracted gonorrhea. These particular trainees were believed to be of very great value to the war effort. However, as Hinds explains, this policy was not without difficulties. During the penicillin program, one man developed an enormous carbuncle that actually appeared to be threatening his life. As his condition worsened, the decision was made to change the man's records (with his permission!) to indicate that he had contracted venereal disease. This done, the penicillin was administered and a rapid recovery followed.

Stories such as these illustrate the way in which new and successful forms of medical care sometimes necessitate triage, especially at first. By the end of World War II, there was enough penicillin to serve the needs of the entire United States armed services and large numbers within the civilian population. But at the time of the early shortages a handful of high-priority patients received the drug while other whose lives might have been saved went without. This same pattern can also be seen with other new developments. For example, the use of the airplane to evacuate the seriously wounded greatly improved the probability of salvaging some casualties. But space on the planes was often very limited, and again triage decisions became essential.

Along with medical treatments that were thought of as almost "miraculous," World War II was the occasion for the development of the most destructive technology known to mankind. The use of nuclear weapons near the end of the war significantly altered the way military triage planners would be able to envision their work in the future. The triage decisions of earlier times were often made in extremely harsh circumstances, but none could compare with the magnitude of the destruction of life and the resources essential to life caused by nuclear weapons. Beebe and DeBakey, prior to their own enunciation of an elaborate triage scheme, describe the changes that must be anticipated now:

> The end of World War II . . . marked the end of an era in military surgery, for the implications of atomic warfare are revolutionary. . . . Planning for atomic warfare must envisage massive obliteration of strategic rear areas, both military and civilian, and must start from an understanding about the responsibility for civilian care. It must contemplate an instantaneous flood of casualties such as no battle ever produced.[35]

Thus, many of the triage systems proposed in military medicine during the 1950s have at least two obvious differences from those of earlier decades. First, such plans must now encompass the civilian population. The cold war and the threat of nuclear attack made this a time for intensive "civil defense" planning with air raid shelters and massive attempts to educate the civilian population about the possibilities for survival. It was also a time for a quantum leap in the numbers of casualties in the contingency-planning scenarios. In the past, triage plans had to include the possibility of as many as 1000 to 2000 casualties being treated in one place at the same time. But now numbers a hundred times larger, and more, must be considered, the larger share of which would be civilians.

A second difference is that during the 1950s triage plans almost always explicitly include distinct categories for those casualties considered either hopeless or too time-consuming. The following summary from a military medical handbook for NATO nations is typical.[36]

1. The slightly injured who can be quickly returned to service
2. The more seriously injured who demand immediate resuscitation or surgery

9

3. The "hopelessly wounded" or dead on arrival

Here, at last, is a "textbook" example of the categories that have come to be widely accepted in military and disaster medicine.

In its section on mass casualties, the handbook cited above clearly states the basic principle upon which this system of triage is founded. After referring to the "sometimes heartbreaking decisions" that must be made, the handbook declares that the military surgeon "must expend his energies in the treatment of only those whose survival seems likely, in line with the objective of military medicine, which has been defined as *'doing the most good for the greatest number* at the proper time and in the proper place.' "[37]

Perhaps enough has now been said about triage in military medicine to permit a few general comments and some analysis before turning to the use of triage in the allocation of new medical therapies.

Hinds has argued that the basis for medical triage has always or nearly always been the medical needs of the patients. In his words:

> When [triage] has been used and where it may be used today
> with a medical connotation, it has meant the allocation of
> priority according to need, and on not other grounds, for goods
> and services in short supply.[38]

But this assertion is incorrect. As has been shown, the principle most often summoned to justify triage in military medicine was the utilitarian principle of the greatest good of the greatest number. This principle was interpreted in at least two distinct ways: 1) the greatest good of the present number of casualties, and 2) the greatest good of the military effort.

Of course, these two applications are not necessarily incompatible. There undoubtedly have been times when preserving military strength was essential to the well-being of the wounded. But in the presentation of these two perspectives it has often been recognized that they may be in conflict, at least in the short run. In the modern discussions of triage in military medicine the goal of maintaining the fighting strength and winning the war increasingly has emerged as the dominant interpretation of the utilitarian principle. This emphasis is seen clearly in the work by Beebe and DeBakey:

Traditionally, the military value of surgery lies in the salvage of battle casualties. This is not merely a matter of saving life; it is *primarily* one of *returning the wounded to duty*, and the earlier the better.[39]

What is almost totally missing in the evolution of triage discussions in military medicine is any mention of justice. Engelhardt is certainly correct when he says, "the use of triage language in wartime medicine often has as its focus winning a war, not attending to the just claims of the persons concerned."[40] This is, of course, hardly surprising. The necessity of military service has often been recognized as an exception to some of the most cherished principles of the social compact of liberal democratic nations. Conscription results in placing the burden of risking life and limb unevenly in the society. This is already a kind of "triage" that in effect sacrifices some "statistical" lives for the sake of the putative good of the larger society. The justification is generally stated in terms of the preservation of the society and not in terms of justice. Thus it does not seem particularly remarkable that triage decisions within military medicine have aimed first of all at achieving those goals for which the military was established.

There is little doubt that with the inception and evolution of triage medical practice had incorporated something new—a structured system of categories for the purpose of making rational decisions about whom to give priority in treatment. It was not long before the triage language of military medicine began to appear in other medical settings.

Triage and New Medical Technologies

It is not hard to find examples of how military medicine has served as a testing ground for many successful new medical therapies and procedures.[41] Mass inoculation techniques, the treatment of infectious diseases, the use of blood plasma and antibiotics, and the development of trauma surgery are but a few examples of areas of medical practice that have been influenced by experience gained in the military. Sorting patients in order to determine priority in treatment is another example.[42]

11

With the lessons about patient sorting learned in the military and with the triage nomenclature and categories fairly well standardized, it was natural that applications be made to the practice of medicine in civilian society. For example, both the word "triage" and some of the criteria for sorting are now commonly used in discussions of mass casualty care[43] and emergency medicine.[44] In these settings it is easy to perceive the relationship of triage to its earlier roots in military medicine. Natural disasters or accidents can and often do result in larger numbers of people needing medical care that might not be immediately available. As with the influx of casualties following a large battle, decisions might be necessary concerning which patients to treat or transport first. Considering the ever-present potential need for such decision making, wisdom and foresight would seem to call for a well-prepared plan of action. The terms and categories of military medicine have provided a starting point for such planning.

In recent years, however, the apparent need for a rational system of sorting and selecting patients has developed in a context far removed from the practice of military, disaster, or emergency medicine. Medical science, in league with modern technology, has created an array of life-saving treatments that are both elaborate and expensive. The production and utilization of these new "high" technologies[45] in medicine have resulted in difficult and largely unforeseen problems of allocation. Probably the most dramatic and widely publicized example occurred in the 1960s with the success of hemodialysis for patients with end-stage renal disease.

The story of patient selection for hemodialysis during the first few years of its availability has been recounted often.[46] There would be no purpose in once again attempting a detailed account here. But certain points deserve emphasis because of their implications for the development of triage thinking in modern medicine.

In the 1940s and 1950s the artificial kidney was in the experimental stages. Hemodialysis of patients with renal failure was usually limited to a few days or weeks at most. The main problem was that each dialysis necessitated a surgery in which tubes were inserted into an artery and a vein, a procedure that could be repeated only a few times.

Then in 1960 Dr. Belding Scribner developed a semipermanent shunt that allowed the patient to be dialyzed on numerous occasions without undergoing a succession of surgeries.[47] This new technique succeeded far beyond Scribner's expectations. It now became possible to keep patients with end-stage renal disease alive for indefinite periods of time.[48] But, as Scribner soon realized, technological achievement was only half a solution.

Almost from the beginning, the success of Scribner's technique caused problems that continued to plague hemodialysis programs for more than a decade and, in fact, are not entirely solved at present. The most obvious and pressing problem can be stated in one word—money. In the 1960s estimates of the cost per year to dialyze one patient in an artificial kidney center ranged from $8000 to $22,000.[49]

Largely because of the cost, but partly because of other factors such as the need for trained personnel, hemodialysis was available for only a very small fraction of the people whose lives potentially could have been saved by the treatment. In order to cut high hospital costs and further the development of dialysis, Scribner and his colleagues were instrumental in establishing the Seattle Artificial Kidney Center at Swedish Hospital in Seattle. But even then they recognized the necessity of setting up some method of patient selection that went beyond the criteria of medical suitability. Consequently, a committee of seven laypersons and physicians, the Admissions and Policy Committee, was appointed by the county's medical association.

The purpose of this committee was to gain support from the community and alleviate the pressure of those in charge of the center by formulating nonmedical criteria for the selection of patients for dialysis.[50] But the policies and procedures generated by the committee resulted in conflict, and in the words of Fox and Swazey, "helped to trigger a lasting and sometimes strident debate about the ethical propriety of such a triage process."[51]

The work of the anonymous committee might have continued to go largely unnoticed had it not been for a feature story written by Shana Alexander for *Life* magazine.[52] Suddenly the committee and its work were thrust before the klieg lights of national scrutiny.

At the time of Alexander's report, the committee had

already selected five patients for dialysis and was preparing to select five more before the year's end. According to the story, the ratio of available places in the dialysis program to the number needing dialysis was about one to fifty. But from the beginning the committee's work was lightened by the fact that medical criteria of exclusion were used to shorten the list of candidates. Some of these criteria were more or less arbitrary. No children were accepted and no patients over forty-five years of age.[53] Prospective candidates were also ruled out if they had other complicating diseases or were deemed psychologically incapable of coping with the treatment regimen.

In addition to the medical criteria of exclusion, the committee decided from the beginning to exclude nonresidents of Washington state. This decision was justified on the grounds that Washington citizens had helped to finance some of the basic research at the University of Washington. The rule automatically eliminated the committee's first candidate, a woman from a neighboring state.[54]

The lawyer on the committee objected to this kind of exclusion. He wondered, for example, if it would not be better to favor a wealthy candidate from another state if such a person would offer to finance treatment for other candidates. As he put it, "[S]pecial attention to one candidate might well work out for the greatest benefit of all."[55] But, he added, "the others couldn't see it that way." As will be seen in a subsequent chapter, the principle of favoring one person in a distribution if this results in added benefits for the others has been defended as just. But the Seattle committee rejected this proposition.

The committee also rejected the idea of casting lots, or random selection. One member commented, "You know, at our committee's first meeting we seriously discussed selecting candidates by drawing straws. We were going to make it easy on ourselves by having a human lottery!"[56] The idea of random selection was repulsive to a majority mostly because it seemed like an irresponsible unwillingness to carry out their appointed task.

That task, as it came to be defined, included a consideration of the patient's "social worth." The rules of preliminary exclusion, including medical, psychological, and geographical factors, so narrowed the field of candidates that the committee had to choose one out of every four rather than the original one out of fifty. It was in selecting the final one from the remaining four that the committee opted for considering criteria of social worth. In the words of one member: "I believe that a man's contribution to society should determine our ultimate decision."[57]

Doubts about their own abilities to determine the relative worth to society of the various candidates were the source of some anxiety. Yet, in spite of the members' willingness to confess their feelings of fallibility, some of them displayed a surprising degree of confidence. For example, the minister reportedly said: "[O]ddly enough, in the choices I have made the correct decision appeared quite clear to me in each case."[58] And the banker commented: "So far, fortunately, we have not had to make a choice between two absolutely equal candidates."[59] He wondered if the physicians were reserving the really tough decisions for a later time when the committee had gained experience.

One may question how the determination of a person's relative social worth could ever be anything like clear-cut. What specific criteria could the committee use that would permit them to have any degree of confidence in the correctness of their decisions? Probably the most often-quoted passage from Alexander's story refers to the factors upon which the committee based its final selections.

> [They] drew up a list of all the factors which they would weigh in making their selection: age and sex of patient; marital status and number of dependents; income; net worth; emotional stability, with particular regard to the patient's capacity to accept the treatment; educational background; nature of occupation, past performance and future potential; and names of people who could serve as references.[60]

Even a brief look at these criteria betrays some of the difficulties encountered in making judgments of social worth. By what calculus can the various factors be computed and evaluated? Is past performance more or less important than future promise? Is wealth a positive or a negative consideration? Do family responsibilities weigh more heavily than contributions to the larger society? Questions such as these could be multiplied indefinitely. Underlying many such questions is

15

a more fundamental concern: Can a selection system based on social worth be fair?

In the debate ignited by the Seattle committee's methods, fairness became a prominent issue. For example, the authors of a law journal article highly critical of the committee's work stated: "[J]ustice requires that selection be made by a fairer method than the unbridled consciences, the built-in biases, and the fantasies of omnipotence of a secret committee."[61] The writers were convinced that an anonymous committee making selections on the basis of an attempted calculation of social worth would surely tend to choose patients who simply mirrored the committee's own value system. Nor were their doubts likely to be alleviated by the comment of one committee member, the labor leader, who indicated that he preferred religious candidates with large families.[62] With such attitudes, the authors argued, the selection process would be virtually certain to favor unfairly the applicants thought to be "respectable" and rule out those considered undesirable, such as nonconformists. In the words of their now famous passage: "The Pacific Northwest is no place for a Henry David Thoreau with bad kidneys."[63]

Sociological research into the outcomes of various selection procedures tended to confirm the charge of class bias. A 1967 survey of eighty-seven artificial kidney centers conducted by Katz and Procter revealed a definite pattern.[64] The majority of selected patients were white (92 percent) married (79 percent) males (75 percent), most of whom were from 35 to 54 years of age. Their education and income levels were somewhat higher than the general population. Indeed, in almost every respect the typical selectee did look like a composite of the Seattle selection comittee, which, to borrow Fox and Swazey's description, was "relatively homogeneous, largely upper middle class in education, occupation, income, and general social background."[65] Six of the seven committee members were also males.

But it must be emphasized that the figures from the survey by Katz and Procter were based on the responses of *eighty-seven* facilities, not just the Seattle center. In only eight of the eighty-seven were lay committees operating at all. And in these eight the committees' functions were not always clear.

The overwhelming majority of centers relied primarily on the physicians to make the final selections. But whether by lay committees or physicians, the pattern of decision making that emerged raised serious questions about the effects of the selectors' personal and social-class biases.

Selection on the basis of social worth was not without its vigorous defenders, however. Shatin, for example, argued that it would be less than honest not to recognize that social values always enter into such a selection process.[66] In his view, such decisions are built on the assumption that "each man occupies a rank within a hierarchy of social value, and this rank determines the amount of medical care or effort which should be expended upon him."[67] With this assumption accepted, Shatin went on to advocate that some rational system for determining criteria of social worth, such as a public survey, be instituted. He rejected as an "extreme thesis" any random selection method, because it might reward the socially disvalued candidates along with their valued counterparts.

In addition to suggesting a public opinion poll, Shatin submitted his own list of social worth considerations. His inventory of ten values included: economic productivity, years of productive life remaining, marital and family status, responsibilities for the welfare of others, medical prognosis, social relationships, potential contributions to society, history of antisocial behavior, and contributions to the "cultural stream of humanity."[68] These factors were not further defined, nor were any instructions given about the relative weight each consideration should receive. Presumably, answers in such matters would be up to the decision-makers. But Shatin failed to identify who such decision-makers should be.

As was already mentioned, the decision-makers in the vast majority of artificial kidney centers were the physicians and not committees of lay persons. This fact was sometimes defended on the grounds that physicians are accustomed to making such decisions. For example, G. E. Schreiner, a prominent physician involved in the development of hemodialysis and transplantation, stated that his institution had no intention of establishing a lay committee to aid in decision making. "We feel that this is a device to spread the responsibility to people who by experience and education are really less

17

equipped to take responsibility than the physicians in charge of the case."[69]

Having pointed out that the medical profession had a long history of making triage decisions, Schreiner suggested that this experience should prove salutary when faced with scarcities of new life-saving remedies. In his words:

> The operational ethical problems facing the dialyser include the concept of triage . . . how we should select patients, and the criteria of selection. However, medicine has been practising triage since the time of Hippocrates. On the battlefield, even with unlimited supplies of blood or albumin, one consciously or subconsciously makes a decision about which person to treat first, usually on the basis of where the most good can be done. The fact that physicians now have to make the choice more deliberately with the uraemic patient does not necessarily make it a totally different problem.[70]

This comment is significant as an indication of the kind of thinking that probably occurred to many practitioners. Triage was *not* new to medicine. Who could possibly be in a better position to make triage decisions than the physicians in charge? And on what better basis could those decisions be made than seeking the "most good" at the time? Schreiner went on to claim that only an "emotional concern about triage" had led to the appointment of lay committees. But he neglected to say just how physicians with their heritage of triage expertise should actually make selections.

Given medicine's long tradition of making triage decisions, one might expect a certain degree of homogeneity in the medical community's approach to patient selection. But such was not the case. Katz and Procter found that variability in applying selection criteria was one of the most striking facts revealed by their study. Even though more than 90 percent of the responding centers reported that physicians were responsible for patient selection, their stated criteria and the methods for applying them were extremely diverse.[71] Some facilities were using social worth criteria that were not divulged to the public, while others openly announced which elements of social worth would be considered. If social worth was weighed, the specific criteria also differed markedly from center to center. Some even went so far as to administer IQ tests, personality inventories, and vocational aptitude tests.[72]

Others relied heavily on the patient's ability to pay for the treatment. Still others made selection on a first-come, first-served basis. And a few were using some random method of selection. Far from finding convergence on the criteria or procedures, researchers found a hodge-podge of approaches. This diversity tended to fuel rather than quell the dispute about the morality of the various systems as advocates defended or condemned one or another selection procedure.

Even as the moral debate about selection was heating, the increased availability of hemodialysis was producing a relaxation in the selection standards. Published reports continued to tell of patients dying for lack of facilities.[73] But as early as 1965 the Seattle center had so expanded its capacity that the Admissions and Policy Committee was seldom called upon to make decisions and for a time was even disbanded.[74]

Then in July 1973 the United States federal government began to subsidize the therapy of patients with end-stage renal disease.[75] Because of the start-up time and the uneven distribution of facilities, however, federal support of hemodialysis did not completely eliminate the need for patient selection. Moreover, there has been a widespread opinion that not all patients with end-stage renal disease are suitable candidates for dialysis even if the facilities have the capacity to treat all of them.[76] Psychological instability or insufficient intelligence, to cite two examples, are factors which have sometimes been considered contraindications for hemodialysis regardless of its availability.

In deciding to subsidize dialysis, the federal government moved the debate about allocation of scarce life-saving resources to a different level. The earlier problems of selecting one patient instead of another are what some have called microallocation decisions.[77] But a national program to support those who suffer from one disease rather than those with some other disease (or all people needing medical care) is what may be called a macroallocation decision. Of this distinction more will be said later. But it is quite obvious that at both the micro- and macroallocation levels triage decisions may be made. At either level, lives may hang in the balance.

Sooner or later, the money spent in one program will usually result in insufficient resources to expand or perhaps even maintain another program. The federal government's renal dialysis program has continued to be plagued by cost overruns and charges of profiteering. And it has become a leading exhibit for those who argue that national health insurance would be a disastrous financial nightmare. Even Dr. Scribner confessed that he has "become deeply troubled over what has happened to my 'brain child.' "[78] Now, almost two decades after Shana Alexander wrote her feature article, the dilemma she articulated seems more pressing than ever:

> Are we moving in the name of science and mercy, toward a nightmare world in which a segment of our population is kept alive by being hooked up to ingenious machines operated by the other half? In such a world the most fit individuals would devote their lives to keeping the least fit alive.[79]

More than any other issue, the debate over dialysis patient selection in general and the decisions of the Seattle committee in particular raised to the level of public consciousness the fact that triage had now become a part of the everyday practice of medicine. Both the term triage and the notion of sorting patients are now referred to as common in medical practice, even in the popular press. A story in one newsmagazine, for example, stated: "Medical resources are in short supply at even the best-equipped of hospitals, and doctors, whether they admit it or not, must perform some sort of triage, or sorting, deciding which patients can be helped and which cannot."[80]

It seems safe to predict that the concept of triage will retain a definite role in medicine for the foreseeable future. Obvious examples of events leading to scarcities and thus to triage include natural disasters and the development of new high technologies. Scarcities such as these may be acute temporarily and then subside.

Other scarcities of medical resources seem to be chronic. But they too may lead to rationing when lives are at stake. For example, in his widely heralded book, *The Gift Relationship*, Titmuss has described the chronic shortages of fresh blood in many urban centers in the United States.[81] In some areas, surgeries have to be scheduled on the basis of available blood supplies. At times the shortages can be life-threatening. The demand for blood in the industrialized nations is rising steadily. But in some countries, such as the United States, the willingness to donate blood has fallen behind the demand. This has led to an expanding international market for human blood and blood derivatives. Not only the blood but also some of its derivatives, such as the clotting factor, are potentially life-saving.[82]

Another well-publicized case in point is the lack of human organs available for transplantation. In Great Britain, for example, the number of people receiving kidney transplants is less than one-fourth of the suitable candidates.[83] Recognition of such shortages has even led some physicians to consider organ procurement as morally obligatory, a fulfillment of a "duty to society."[84]

A final example is the shortage of trained medical personnel in some geographical areas. In the developed nations the problem is usually one of maldistribution of the available personnel.[85] In most instances the difficulties encountered in attempting to see a physician, such as the extra distance traveled, are not life-threatening. But the relative isolation of some communities can make the absence of trained medical personnel a serious problem.

Summary and Conclusion

Triage has now become an integral part of present-day medicine not only in its more "exotic" forms with high technologies but sometimes even in the more common practices of everyday medical care. The sterile operating rooms and hushed halls of a modern medical facility seem exceedingly far removed from the din of a World War I battle. But triage has played an important role in such widely divergent contexts. As the nuances of the concept of triage have evolved, certain elements have remained relatively constant; others have not.

For the purposes of this discussion, an important continuity is the dominant type of justification that generally has been given for triage. When a reason has been stated, it has been usually in terms of doing the greatest good for the greatest number. This principle is implied, for example, when the decision is made to leave aside an especially time-consuming patient if several others might be treated in the same time period. The principle is also at work in the use of social worth

21

criteria to select patients for renal dialysis. It is only slightly less evident in the medical, psychological, and sociological screenings that have preceded the application of social worth criteria in selecting dialysis candidates. The principle obviously has a strong intuitive appeal in triage situations. What could seem more reasonable than "making the best" of otherwise tragic circumstances? Moreover, appealing to the utilitarian principle receives hefty support from the prevailing moral spirit of the age. One or another brand of utilitarianism has tended to dominate moral thought in modern times.

And yet, one of the most obvious discontinuities in the development of medical triage stems from the ambiguity of this prevailing justificatory principle. In both military and civilian medicine, triage for the "greatest good" has sometimes meant attempting to minimize the harm for the largest possible number of patients and sometimes seeking to maximize the good for some larger cause or reference group such as the military effort, the patients' families, or even the entire society. Thus, the triage process raises fundamental questions about justice. If the amplitude of life-saving or life-supporting resources is insufficient to serve all who are in need, should the utilitarian approach be considered just? If so, for whom should the harm be minimized or the good maximized? For the patients? For the society as a whole? Are there other approaches that better match our studied convictions about justice? Or do the dire scarcities of triage situations obviate all principles of justice?

It is clear that when Larrey initiated his "methodical" scheme for rationing medical care on the battlefield, he prided himself in treating the wounded strictly on the basis of medical need without regard for rank or distinction. But, as we have now seen, this essentially egalitarian approach gave way to a variety of schemes based primarily on utilitarian considerations. No one is known to have challenged the justice of the utilitarian approaches to triage in *military* or *emergency* medicine.[86] In fact, even general questions concerning the morality of military or disaster triage are almost never discussed.[87] Serious challenges have been mounted, however, against utilitarian approaches to triage in civilian medicine, especially in the allocation of high technologies. Proponents of a more

22

strictly egalitarian approach to triage, reminiscent of Larrey's rationing on the basis of medical needs, have raised their voices in protest and started a long and sometimes heated debate.

These developments suggest some puzzling questions. Why do applications of utilitarian reasoning which seem to go unchallenged in one context bring forth vigorous egalitarian objections in another? What are the morally relevant differences, if any, in the different settings? In order to pursue these questions further, I now turn to an analysis of two cases in which triage planning is already being discussed for situations that are still in the future.

II Two Prismatic Cases

THE TWO CASES DISCUSSED in this chapter have been chosen for their "prismatic" qualities.[1] Although they illustrate to some extent the usual factors that might be expected as a part of triage planning in modern medicine, they can hardly be called typical. They are not garden-variety examples selected from a large number of similar instances. Rather they have been picked because they permit an analysis of some of the salient elements that affect triage decision making. What is more, these cases show the spectrum of morally relevant features that constitute the moral dilemma of triage.

The two cases are the contingency planning for the next major earthquake in San Francisco and the discussions about the development and allocation of totally implantable artificial hearts. In both instances, deliberations about triage are already taking place for circumstances that have not yet occurred. The fact that both events are still in the future may make it seem strange to refer to them as cases. Does it make sense to discuss a case that has not yet transpired and may never come to pass? The answer, of course, is that the main concern here is not for the actual events, which at this point may be discussed only hypothetically (or "futuristically," to borrow recent usage). Rather, of far greater importance for this discussion are the kinds of factors that affect triage planning, the alternatives being considered, and the supporting reasons being given. Thus, in what follows, the cases under scrutiny are the *deliberations* about the conduct of triage during the anticipated events.

24

Triage Planning for a San Francisco Earthquake

The director of San Francisco's Office of Emergency Services has the unenviable task of preparing contingency plans for a dreaded event.[2] One wag has dubbed him "Chancellor of the Apocalypse."[3] An important part of his role is to coordinate the efforts of numerous institutions and government agencies in developing plans to cope with the next major San Francisco earthquake.

According to estimates in the city's earthquake response plan, a quake the magnitude of the one in 1906 could cause more than 10,000 deaths and more than 40,000 injuries requiring hospitalization.[4] The casualties would result not only from the immediate effects of the quake, such as falling glass and masonry and the collapse of buildings, but also from the subsequent fires and flash floods. In some instances, these secondary effects would be more destructive than the initial earthquake. For example, many of the communities in the Bay Area are located in potential inundation tracts just below dams or reservoirs.[5]

Attempts to aid the injured and rescue the trapped are likely to be multiplied by the threat of fire. Numerous fires, some very extensive, are expected to burn out of control. Because of broken water lines and impassable streets, fighting the fires would be difficult if not impossible. And the amount of water in the emergency cisterns would be insufficient to control the large number of fires that are anticipated.

The projected ability to care for the tens of thousands of casualties is not reassuring. The actual number of casualties would likely vary a great deal depending on the time of day at which the earthquake would occur. The estimates of 30,000 to 40,000 casualties, the figures given in the current Earthquake Response Plan, are considered far too low by some observers.[6] In any event, the medical needs of the enormous number of injured people would almost certainly surpass the available medical resources. For example, after sustaining major quake damage, the available hospital beds are likely to be less than half the number needed. Shortages of other medical resources could be even more detrimental to life-saving efforts. For example, the city has approximately forty-six ambulances, including both government and privately owned vehicles.[7] But most of the ambulances that still would be operative after a quake would be used as aid stations, not to transport casualties. Buses, taxis, and other available transportation would carry some of the injured, but the small number of usable vehicles and the impassability of many streets would greatly hamper the movement of casualties.

The number of medical personnel may also be inadequate. Here again the degree of scarcity would depend largely on the time of the earthquake. The city has a high concentration of medical personnel. But a large percentage of these persons live outside the city and would not be immediately available during much of the twenty-four-hour day. And many of the medical personnel within the city at the time of an earthquake would themselves become casualties.

A list of other scarcities of medical resources would no doubt include such items as drugs, whole blood, and the electrical power to operate medical devices such as respirators. The official response plan summarizes the anticipated difficulties:

> The shortage of [hospital] beds, coupled with the loss and damage to facilities and equipment, loss of medical supplies, deaths and injuries to doctors, nurses and technical personnel, and difficulties in obtaining required power, constitutes [sic] significant problems in the area of emergency medical assistance.[8]

In view of the uncertainties about the extent of the potential damage, the time of day and year, and a host of other complexities, it is not hard to imagine the inordinate difficulty of preparing rational response strategies. But it is the responsibility of the Office of Emergency Services (OES) to develop and continually update just such a plan.

At the heart of this planning is the division of the city into four zones.[9] The main part of the city, Zone Four, is then subdivided into ten districts, roughly paralleling the ten fire districts used by the fire department under normal operating conditions. In the event of a major earthquake, the fire battalion chief in each of the ten districts would become the director of emergency services in that particular district. The fire department would bear the brunt of the responsibility for preserving order and initiating aid and rescue responses, including triage.

According to the OES plan, the first sorting of casualties and administration of first aid would take place at a "Casualty Care Facility" reminiscent of the World War I Casualty Clearing Stations. The official response plan calls for the personnel at this facility to perform "triage (the process of sorting the injured on the basis of urgency and type of condition presented so that they can be properly routed to medical care)."[10] The plan indicates that "triage teams" based in several of the hospitals should be dispatched to the Casualty Care Facilities after initial reconnaisance has been completed. These teams are responsible for the advanced triage planning. But it is probably wishful thinking to expect all Casualty Care Facilities to be staffed by medically trained triage teams. In the words of one OES document: "Field treatment will need to be accomplished in many cases by non-medical or para-medical personnel."[11]

Because of the anticipated difficulties in conducting triage, there are doubts about its effectiveness, especially in the first minutes following a major quake. In the words of one planner: "Triage doesn't always work. No matter how well rigged you are, the trend is to send to the hospital the people you get out first, no matter how slightly or severely injured they are."[12] But the official quickly added that as conditions gradually stabilized, the number of casualties at the various facilities would almost certainly exceed the available resources, and triage would become necessary.

The goal of triage is stated in one OES document: "Optimizing the use of [the available medical] resources in response to a major emergency or disaster is expected to prevent or minimize loss of life, disabling injuries or pain and discomfort."[13] Making optimal use of medical resources in order to minimize harm is clearly reflected in the proposed use of triage. Thus, the treatment of casualties deemed hopeless would be considered an unacceptable waste of time. It is also generally agreed that priority should be given to those with medical competence, so that their skills could be put to use aiding the others in need. As one planner put it, "Priority should definitely be given to those with special skills such as medical personnel."[14]

The response plans are also clear about why priorities must be set if greater harm is to be avoided. "Everything cannot be done that should be done, considering the limitations of both time and resources."[15] Thus, scarcity leads to triage—not only the scarcity of material resources but also the shortages of time and energy and skills.

Triage and the Artificial Heart

The 1976 report of the President's Biomedical Research Panel revealed both the hope and the apprehension generated by the prospect of a successful totally implantable artificial heart (TIAH).[16] For tens of thousands of Americans who suffer from serious heart disease, the nation's leading cause of death, TIAH offers the hope of longer, more productive lives. Although that hope may seem remote, the panel's report included the prediction that the first version of a working TIAH for human beings "will become available well before the turn of the century."[17] And more recent reports indicate that TIAH will become a clinical reality in the 1980s.[18] But the panel also wondered about society's ability to cope with such a development.

According to the report, the number of prospective recipients of TIAH would be on the order of ten times as large as those requiring hemodialysis. Even though the maintenance costs for TIAH recipients probably will be much less than those for dialysis patients, the initial costs for TIAH and its implantation are likely to be many times higher. Will society be willing to pay the bill for all who need TIAH? Will there be a sufficient number of surgeons who are competent to perform the intricate implantation procedures? The report did not suggest solutions for such problems, which it calls "extraordinarily difficult."[19]

The idea of an artificial heart is not new. In 1939 John H. Gibbon was able to keep cats alive for almost three hours by using a mechanical substitute for both heart and lungs.[20] And as early as 1948 the National Heart and Lung Institute (NHLI) was funding research on various kinds of circulatory assist devices. With the development of cardiovascular surgery, especially in the 1950s, interest in mechanical heart and lung machines was greatly intensified.

By the mid-1950s several researchers had begun to give serious attention to the development of TIAH.[21] Such a mechanical heart, it was hoped, would avoid the problems of the patient's dependency on external support systems and the anticipated problems of incompatibility associated with transplant therapy. The development of TIAH received a major boost in 1964 when the United States Congress approved allocations specifically designated for research on the artificial heart. The funding resulted in the establishment of the Artificial Heart Program Office. Since then, the program has continued to receive funding at an annual rate of several million dollars.[22] And research has produced definite improvements in artificial heart technology.

Work on TIAH has not been limited to the United States. Other countries, such as Japan and West Germany, have vigorous research programs.[23] And since 1974, the United States has participated in a joint research and development program with the Soviet Union.[24] This program, headed by Dr. Michael DeBakey, has fostered an exchange of information and devices.

But despite the concerted efforts of numerous investigators and the sponsorship of governments and private industry, TIAH is still beset by some serious technical problems.[25] For example, none of the various energy sources for TIAH is free of difficulties. Conventional batteries must be recharged and eventually replaced, and nuclear energy sources may give off harmful radiation. The search also continues for an elastic material that can ensure the millions of contractions and expansions necessary for proper heart function in even the period of one year.[26] Among the difficult problems facing TIAH researchers at present are the device's tendencies to destroy blood cells and cause clotting.[27] But progress continues to be made in the search for materials that do not harm the blood and to eliminate areas of turbulence and stagnation in the flow of blood.[28]

Progress toward solutions of TIAH's problems is being made

steadily. Only a few years ago, keeping a calf alive with an implanted artificial heart for a few hours to a few days was considered a major success. Now, reports of such test animals being kept alive for several months are becoming more frequent.[29]

The technical problems associated with TIAH show every sign of being resolvable. But questions about the potential social, economic, and ethical ramifications continue to be raised. Dr. Belding Scribner has admonished the developers of TIAH and other high medical technologies to recognize that technical success is "just halfway" to the goal; problems of scarcity and adequate funding must also be faced.[30] At the end of its statement on the artificial heart, the President's Biomedical Research Panel recommended that "serious research efforts" be made in an attempt to predict and assess the social and economic consequences of the anticipated success of TIAH.

However, such an attempt already has been made. In the summer of 1972 NHLI assembled an interdisciplinary group of highly respected scholars for the purpose of evaluating the potential effects of TIAH.[31] The Artificial Heart Assessment Panel held regular meetings from September 1972 to May 1973 in order to carry out its charge "to present a report detailing the economic, ethical, legal, medical, psychiatric, and social implications" of the clinical use of TIAH.[32]

The panel, made up largely of members with nonmedical backgrounds, undertook an unprecedented venture. Indeed, the entire idea of attempting to assess the social impact of new technology was quite new. Small wonder, then, that the panel expressed dismay at the short period of time allocated for the preparation of its report.[33] Nevertheless, in June 1973 the panel submitted its work, which was subsequently published.

The report conveyed a generally positive attitude toward the development of TIAH. It was admitted that the panel had initially thought of the potential advent of TIAH as an "earth-shaking event." But gradually and "somewhat reluctantly" TIAH came to be viewed as similar to "other major medical innovations."[34] Much of the panel's work was devoted to analyzing the potential cost and benefits of TIAH. In the panel's view, the hoped-for benefits clearly superseded the potential costs. In the words of the report: "If all of the expectations of its sponsors are realized, its benefits to society will be immense."[35]

Although much of the report was devoted to the kind of cost/benefit analysis often associated with utilitarian decisions, the panel was reluctant to rely exclusively on this type of reasoning. In the panel's judgment, the fact that some members of society might be exposed to additional risk, even though statistically insignificant,[36] was sufficient reason to caution against the use of plutonium 238 as a power source for TIAH. It was recognized that the use of a nuclear power source might eventually bring great benefits to a very large number of recipients while at the same time only increasing the chances of genetic defects or death due to such causes as cancer and leukemia by a very small factor. But for the majority of panel members the utilitarian justification that would permit the genetic damage or death of a few people in order to provide the benefits of a nuclear-powered TIAH for many people was morally unacceptable. In their words: "While critics have noted many defects in the utilitarian philosophy, the defect of most concern to the Panel is the lack of clarity about distribution of benefits and burdens in a manner consonant with justice and fairness."[37]

The panel admitted that it could not "solve the theoretical problems of utilitarianism and justice."[38] But the majority of the members were convinced that the utilitarian principle of the greatest good for the greatest number was an inadequate basis for approaching many of the moral questions raised by TIAH.[39] Distributive justice, they concluded, was not simply a matter of making good-maximizing decisions. Other principles, such as equality of access to the good and adequate compensation for the disadvantaged "lesser number," must be taken into account. The panel's concern for fairness is particularly obvious in the deliberations and conclusions about the problems of allocating a potentially scarce life-saving resource.

It is probable that for some time after clinical trials have successfully demonstrated the effectiveness of TIAH, various kinds of scarcities will be encountered. Thus, it is likely that for some period of time a large number of patients who need and want the devices will find them unavailable. At one time or another, such shortages would probably include not only the artificial hearts but also medical personnel who are competent to implant the devices and adequate power sources to run the devices. And, as with the earlier development of renal dialysis, the most difficult scarcity to overcome may be that of money.

Even in 1973, the estimated cost of one TIAH (including implantation and associated medical care) ran as high as $25,000 and the estimated number of potential recipients was as many as 50,000.[40] This means that the costs to society, if the political decisions to bear those costs were made, could be far in excess of one billion dollars each year. And it must not be forgotten that this projection is based on 1973 estimates. Judging from the experience with renal dialysis, it may take the society a considerable length of time to make the commitment to provide TIAH for all who are in need.

Partly because the development of TIAH has been and will continue to be supported by public funds, the Artificial Heart Assessment Panel recommended that any successful device "should be broadly available, and availability should not be limited only to those able to pay."[41] But the panel recognized that even with adequate funds, other factors could cause shortages. Thus, anticipating various kinds of scarcities, the panel addressed itself to the problems of allocation.

Three alternative methods of rationing were considered: (1) selection on the basis of medical need, (2) selection on the basis of social worth, and (3) selection on the basis of some random method. The panel concluded that in conditions of scarcity patients should be chosen first and foremost on the basis of medical need. "Under such a system," the panel said, "a medical center would determine, strictly on medical criteria, which of the candidate patients being treated by the medical center have the greatest need for implantation of the artificial heart and are suitable candidates (e.g., can withstand the trauma of surgery, etc.)."[42]

The panel's interpretation of the criterion of medical needs reveals two important considerations: the severity of the patient's medical condition and the probability of a successful implantation. It seems clear that these would be countervailing factors in the cases of some patients. At some point, for example, the patient's physical deterioration probably would begin to reduce the chances of successful implantation. Presumably, therefore, decisions based on the urgency of medical need and the probability of success would be highly technical exercises in balancing complex medical considerations. Such decisions would seem to require the abilities of skilled medical personnel.

But what should happen if expert analyses of the candidates' medical conditions resulted in a list of equally needy and suitable prospective recipients? The panel decided that candidates with "roughly equivalent" medical needs should be selected by some random method. Such a random selection, the panel indicated, "could be implemented either by lottery or by a system of first-come first-served."[43] It is important to notice that the system of first-come, first-served is apparently equated with a lottery, with both being seen as types of random selection.

Much of the panel's discussion of patient selection was devoted to a consideration of selection on the basis of social worth criteria. The report said that a "persuasive case" could be made for the position that society is justified in saving its more exemplary or productive members. The panel agreed that social worth criteria do tend to affect medical decision making much of the time. Would it not be more honest to recognize this fact and subject such criteria to public scrutiny? Persuasive as the logic may seem, the majority of panel members remained unconvinced.

The panel pointed out the difficulties in establishing fair and workable social worth criteria: people are usually unwilling to make the tough decisions required, general agreement on such criteria seems unobtainable, and it would be virtually impossible to apply the criteria in an "even handed and objective manner."[44] The report went on to say that "the very essence of making decisions based on 'social worth' runs counter to basic principles of equality in our society."[45] In the end the idea of selection on the basis of social worth was totally rejected.

Rejected, that is, by *nearly* all the panel members. Clark

Havighurst, professor of law at Duke University, disagreed. In a long appendix, he criticized the panel for its failure to develop a "coherent conceptual framework."[46] Havighurst agreed that complete reliance on a utilitarian weighing of benefits and costs would be ethically unacceptable. But in his view, a more adequate model would be "the economist's perfect world, in which all interactions are costless and all conflicts among individuals can therefore be resolved in voluntary transactions rather than through governmental intervention."[47]

Even a long appendix leaves the reader somewhat uncertain about the full implications of Havighurst's position. But the view that seems to emerge is a kind of utilitarianism tempered by a strong concern for losers in various social interactions. According to Havighurst, this concern for losers does not mean that the prospect of a few uncompensated losers overrules a particular decision. After all, he argues, failure to pursue a project that would result in net benefits would be a kind of harm to those who might otherwise have been "winners." Nevertheless, compensation to the losers should be provided whenever possible.

Using this model, Havighurst arrived at conclusions about patient selection which were sometimes different from those of the majority of the panel members. He criticized the panel's report for its "superficiality," and he linked the questions of patient selection to the problems of financing TIAH. Havighurst challenged the notion that the high technologies of modern medicine must be provided for all members of society. He wondered what point there would be in providing the poor with high-cost therapies such as TIAH when more basic kinds of medical care are not supplied. He also questioned the advisability of having the government involved in triage. He apparently felt that if the government were given the role of triage decision making, society's humanitarian image would be tarnished. He asked:

> [I]n which of the following cases is the government more (least) deeply implicated in a human death: When it occurs because a legislatively set benefit is exceeded? When charitable resources, available for some, are not made available in a particular case? When a publicly established selection system, random or otherwise, turns the patient

down? When, even though the patient was able to pay from his private resources or from insurance which he had purchased a public selection process gave the only available treatment to a patient whose treatment was supported by the taxpayers? When a large side payment, or the physician's perception of social worth, leads to preferring one patient over another who is poorer or less socially prominent?[48]

It may be that Havighurst considered some of the selection systems mentioned in these questions to be fairer than others. But fairness was not his main concern; government responsibility was. And on this point, he made it clear that he favored those approaches that would limit government's role and rely more heavily on charity.

Havighurst took special pains to criticize the panel for its failure to treat the questions of macroallocation carefully. In the report the majority of the panel members expressed the view that society's putative commitment to save every possible life is at best a valuable myth.[49] Such a myth might be needed in order to preserve certain social values, but it hardly could be considered a true representation of the facts. But, Havighurst complained, the panel went on to accept the inevitability of TIAH without seriously questioning whether or not the money could be spent to greater advantage on other kinds of programs. In Havighurst's view, assuaging society's conscience by providing high technologies like TIAH is of dubious value. He argued that "unlimited government financing will call forth many more expensive technologies."[50]

Whether or not Havighurst was right in this prediction, he was correct in saying that the report did not include any extensive discussion of macroallocation decisions. Why should heart disease take precedence over numerous other catastrophic diseases? What limits should be set on research or subsidization of medical care for any one category of diseases? These and other macroallocation questions are exceedingly difficult, perhaps impossible, to answer. But neither their inordinate complexity nor their tendency to affect "statistical" lives rather than clearly identifiable individuals can alter the fact that macroallocation decisions often represent a kind of rationing or triage, and thus deserve scrutiny from the perspective of distributive justice.[51] Because these decisions are ultimately political decisions, and because they affect a large segment of the society, they deserve to be aired as widely as possible. As Albert Jonsen has written in his own analysis of the panel's work: "Problems of distributive justice, which this development [of TIAH] raises in a vivid way, must be debated in the public forum."[52]

Reflections on the Cases

The brief presentation of these two cases permits some further observations about the nature of triage. The cases obviously represent vastly different contexts, and many of the differences will become even more obvious in the chapters that follow as the moral significance of the dissimilarities is explored. But it should be noted at this point that the cases also reveal common elements of medical triage of which the following are some of the more prominent:

1. There must be a scarcity of some life-saving medical resource.

2. The scarcity of medical resources must be *obvious*. Unless the amplitude of the life-saving medical resource in question is clearly insufficient, triage probably would not take place. If the resource appears to be nearly adequate or if there is much uncertainty about its sufficiency, then it is likely that patients would be treated primarily on a first-come, first-served basis.

3. The shortage must be expected to continue for some (indefinite) period of time. If the scarce resources are readily and immediately expandable, it would again seem likely that people would attempt to "make do," without attempting to establish a rational system or patient selection. For example, a significant factor in the triage planning for a San Francisco earthquake is the likelihood that the city would become relatively isolated for a time, and adequate relief supplies would not be immediately available.

4. Triage requires order, including the establishment of some authority. In his description of what a San Francisco earthquake might be like, Koughan says: "Warnings against looting are disregarded; people fight for scarce medical supplies, blankets, and food."[53] If this scenario is realistic (and who

knows for sure?), then triage would be impossible. The people who are formulating San Francisco's earthquake contingency plans hope that fire and police personnel will be able to maintain or reestablish order. But without such authority figures whose legitimacy is widely accepted, the order necessary for triage probably would be lacking.

The anticipated allocation of artificial hearts reveals another aspect of the need for authority. The expert opinions of medical personnel would be necessary in order to conduct rationing. Not only must the medical need of the candidates be ascertained, but also the chances for success must be predicted. Obviously, the authority of medical personnel would be essential.

5. Planning for triage is complex, difficult, and sometimes impossible. It might seem that most of the scarcities necessitating triage could be eliminated through careful planning. But the fact that this is often impossible is demonstrated by the two cases under discussion. For example, with the knowledge currently available, the precise location, the magnitude, and many other aspects of San Francisco's next earthquake cannot be fully predicted. Thus triage planning must proceed with a very large factor of uncertainty.

Likewise, the future of TIAH is uncertain. TIAH may never be a success, or the first successful clinical trials may come very soon. There is no way to make preparations for mass production of a device that still must be modified extensively. Moreover, it is impossible to train medical personnel to do procedures that have not yet been tested. As the President's Biomedical Research Panel asked in its discussion of TIAH: "[H]ow does one prepare ahead of time to provide people with the skills to carry out this type of surgery?"[54]

6. Triage planning and decisions are affected by the availability of money. The effects of macroallocation decisions can hardly be ignored in a discussion of triage planning and administration. Lack of funds can result in the shortages of medical resources that make triage necessary, as may be seen eventually with TIAH.

7. Triage decisions may involve the distribution of huge burdens as well as the most basic of benefits, the means to continue life. In his recent book on artificial organs, Kolff

describes research that is continuing to demonstrate the advantages of a nuclear-powered TIAH.[55] If, as now seems likely, such research results in successful devices implanted in some recipients, it is highly probable that the other members of society will have accepted (or been given) some enormous burdens. The risks of radiation, including the increased probability of cancer and genetic damage, have already been mentioned. The nuclear power source also is likely to be very expensive. Kolff indicates that the most successful nuclear-driven engine currently available uses sixty grams of plutonium 238, at a cost of about $1000 per gram. And, he adds, this is a savings of $20,000 or more over other nuclear-powered versions! Without some type of insurance, it is obvious that the use of such devices would be limited to the wealthier members of society.

Some of the burdens distributed by triage decisions are not as measurable as the dollar costs. There are, for example, the psychological burdens that must be borne by those who are not selected and by their families. There are the burdens of uncertainty and anguish that must be accepted by the decision-makers (at least if they are sensitive). In numerous and often subtle ways, triage calls for sacrifices, including the loss of life for some, so that others may go on living.

Because triage decisions involve the allocation of important burdens and benefits, it might seem indisputable that the fairness of such decisions should be considered. Offhand, it would appear incontrovertible that triage raises questions about distributive justice. But the matter is far from settled. Numerous authors have argued that *no* principle of distributive justice is applicable in the situations of dire scarcity that necessitate triage. These arguments and an attempt to resolve them are discussed in the next chapter.

III Dire Scarcity and Distributive Justice

THE PROBLEM DISCUSSED in this chapter is presented nicely by Nicholas Rescher: "An *economy of scarcity* is, by definition, one in which justice (in the restricted sense of the term) cannot be done, because there is not 'enough to go around. . . .'"[1] At what point, if any, does justice become impossible when scarcity is encountered? This is the question that must now be addressed.

The Concept of Dire Scarcity

The inability to produce enough goods to satisfy human desires is *the* economic problem. During the 1970s the realities of overpopulation and famine on the one hand and overconsumption on the other have painfully reminded us of a perennial aspect of human experience, the need to economize. Now, perhaps even more than in the past, it is necessary to think carefully about the concept of scarcity and its implications for moral responsibility.

However, the concept of scarcity can be deceptively difficult to analyze. Like other relative concepts, such as "relative poverty," scarcity presents certain conceptual problems. The basic idea of scarcity is easy enough to grasp: the amount of some good (or the means for attaining it) is insufficient to satisfy the desires of all who want such a good. But embedded in this apparently simple notion are complexities, some of which have important bearing on our discussion of triage and distributive justice.

It is important to notice, for instance, that the concept of scarcity refers not only to relative *amounts* of some item, but also to relative *levels of desirability*. Even if only one mosquito arrives at a picnic, it is unlikely that anyone will speak of a scarcity of mosquitos. Concern about a shortage of sandwiches or cake is far more probable. Thus, to say that something is scarce usually means that it is valued; at least some people have reasons to want it.

This relationship of desirability to scarcity can be observed with regard to medical resources. For example, Dr. Lewis Thomas has argued that the artificial heart is an "essentially hideous engine."[2] According to Thomas, TIAH is "halfway technology" that is expensive, undesirable, and likely to become an "instant antique" as soon as a solution to coronary artery disease can be found. For Thomas and those who agree with him, even a few artificial hearts would be too many.

Of course, if everyone agreed with Thomas, TIAH would not be developed (unless as part of some sinister plot). But the fact is that many people would find a clinically acceptable TIAH to be highly desirable, especially when compared to the prospects of almost certain death without the device. For these people, the availability of only a few artificial hearts would be perceived as a case of extreme scarcity. The difference between Thomas and the people who desire TIAH is at least partly one of values. Such differences in the kinds of things people value are often fortunate, else the problems occasioned by many scarcities would be greatly exacerbated. The diversity of human desires tends to distribute demands and lessen the severity of some shortages.

However, another feature of the relationship between desirability and scarcity is the fact that most goods that can be called scarce are wanted by more than one person. It is not impossible to think of cases in which only one person would have reasons to want some scarce good (for example, one person stranded on an island with an inadequate supply of fresh water). But such cases are exceptional. To say that some good is in short supply nearly always means that a number of people desire it and are competing for it.

In addition to the relationship between scarcity and desires, it is also important to discuss some of the difficulties posed by the distinction between *needs* and desires. Perhaps a discussion of triage could justifiably ignore this problem on the grounds that the goods in question are, by definition, necessary for the preservation of life. The more basic the needs, the more likely it would seem that needs and desires would converge. For example, if we consider Maslow's well-known "hierarchy of needs," we see that the physiological needs are referred to as the most basic.[3] It is precisely this kind of basic need that the resources allocated in triage are capable of satisfying. Thus, anyone who had such a need could be expected to desire the means for satisfying it. Life-supporting medical resources probably would be included in any list of goods that, to borrow an expression from Rawls, a person may be assumed to "want whatever else he wants."[4]

However, this does not mean that the problem of "false needs" can be ignored completely.[5] It is not impossible that people could be convinced (for example, through some sort of manipulative advertising) to feel a need for "life-saving" remedies that may, in fact, be of dubious value in that they are ineffective or entail very undesirable side effects. Even at the level of what appear to be the most basic needs, a system of values is clearly at work. As Barry has argued, to say that "A needs X" is usually an incomplete way of saying that "A needs X to do Y."[6] The in-order-to portion of the statement is usually unnecessary because it is obvious to the hearer by implication. Thus to say "A needs an artificial heart" probably implies the ending "in order to continue life." Stated negatively, we may say that A needs an artificial heart to avoid the harm of further suffering or death.

This negative form of the statement illustrates an important part of the relationship of the concepts of scarcity and needs. The need that A has for X could be called false if not obtaining X would result in *no* further *harm* to A.[7] Thus, when we assert "A needs X," we usually are considering the probable harm that will be sustained by A if X is not acquired. For example, to say "A needs a blood transfusion" means that without the transfusion A will suffer further harm. It is clear that A might not always *desire* what is needed (for example, if A were unconscious or in shock). It is also clear that if the blood transfusion would bring more harm to A than no transfusion (for example, if the blood were contaminated with a deadly disease or poison), then it would make no sense to say that A needed that

41

particular transfusion. Or, to take the example of the artificial heart, in order to claim that a potential recipient would not need such a device, it would be necessary to show that the harm caused by it would be greater than the harm of not having it implanted.

The evaluation of such potential outcomes would certainly require special knowledge about the patient's condition and the relevant statistical probabilities. But a strong case can be made for leaving the final decision to the patient, insofar as that is possible.[8] In most cases, it would seem that the patient is the one best able to determine which course of action would represent the least harm from the perspective of his/her own life plan. The Artificial Heart Assessment Panel expressed this view by stating:

> The Panel believes that decisions about the quality of life with an artificial heart are essentially personal and that, to the greatest extent possible, decisions concerning implantation should be made by the patient himself and not by physicians, who may be tempted to believe that they are able adequately to appraise the patient's interests.[9]

Let us summarize the argument thus far: When we say that a resource is both *scarce* and *needed*, we mean that some people will probably suffer harm because of the shortage. Although the prediction of potential harm (and thus the determination of need) is often a complex matter, the decision belongs ultimately to the one who must personally bear the results.

Two other aspects of the concept of scarcity must be examined. First, to say that something is scarce often depends on the expectations of those who have reasons to desire the resource. In the 1950s, moon rocks were not thought of as scarce. But, following the Apollo space missions, a few pounds of moon rocks became available. Now, from the perspective of interested scientists, the rocks seem very scarce. Similarly, because no workable artificial heart has yet been developed, it seems inappropriate to speak of scarcity. However, if *one* successful artificial heart becomes available, the conditions of extreme scarcity would appear to have been "created." Offhand, this seems to be one of the odd features of the concept of scarcity. It seems strange that in moving from no resources to a few resources the sense of scarcity may be heightened (one might even say originated). But the explanation of this apparent oddity is the change from a state of wishful thinking to a state of actual possibility. Once the needed item becomes available to anyone, the expectations of others in need may be fostered. This does not mean that a person who might need the resource must have "high" expectations of receiving it, but it does mean that the resource must be at least remotely capable of being obtained, people must know that it exists, and they must know that it is beneficial.

The final characteristic of scarcity that deserves attention has to do with the divisibility of the resource in question. Some scarce resources can be divided and subdivided into smaller and smaller portions. The smaller amounts may be less effective and yet still be better than nothing. An example of a medical resource of this divisible type is the hormone used to stimulate growth in children who would otherwise suffer from dwarfism. According to Dr. Raymond Hintz of Stanford University, the demand for the hormone greatly exceeds the available supply.[10] Because of the scarcity, only a small percentage of the children who need the hormone can be treated. Children are allowed to stay in the treatment program only until they have reached a height of five feet. In this example, the amount of benefit to be given to any one recipient can be determined largely in advance because of the divisibility of the resource.

But many goods and services, including medical resources, obviously cannot be divided and still be effective. One artificial heart cannot be shared by several recipients. And the divisibility of other resources is often very limited. For example, the available time on a kidney machine can be shared only by a limited number of dialysis patients. Beyond this limit, an attempt to share the machine with more patients probably would result in earlier deaths for all the patients.

The limited divisibility of a scarce resource is an important part of what I shall call *dire scarcity*.[11] On the basis of the preceding analysis, the circumstances of dire scarcity can be described as follows: The amount of some life-saving resource, which cannot be further divided without losing its life-saving capacity, is insufficient to sustain the lives of all who are in need. These circumstances must be distinguished from those of *moderate scarcity*. Under the conditions of moderate scarcity, the goods in question may be divided so that everyone who has a claim may receive a share roughly equivalent to his or her claim. Here, the division is in terms of "more or less." But under the conditions of dire scarcity, a good that is needed to sustain life cannot be provided to all who need it, no matter what their claims may be. Here, the only possible distribution must be in terms of "all or nothing." These are the conditions that lead to triage. And, according to some writers, these same circumstances make justice impossible.

Dire Scarcity and the Possibility of Justice

One of the most widely accepted tenets of moral philosophy is that "ought implies can."[12] It seems nonsensical to say that a person ought to have done something that clearly was impossible. One can only be praised or blamed for doing or failing to do that which was within his or her power to accomplish. It follows that any scarcity can affect our judgment of moral obligation to the extent that such scarcity hinders the action of the moral agent.

This point has been discussed at considerable length by Vivian Charles Walsh in his book, *Scarcity and Evil*. Walsh writes: "There is no property except blamelessness that the effects of scarcity cannot destroy."[13] Ascriptions of moral responsibility, Walsh argues, are often mistaken because the subtle effects of scarcity are not considered. Scarcity is not just an isolated part of experience. Rather, it is the pervasive economic aspect of all human existence. The means that are necessary to accomplish desired ends are often in short supply. The ends are often in competition. Thus, even the person of consistently good will is frequently prevented from carrying out the dictates of that will.

All of this may seem perfectly obvious. But Walsh claims that many deeds which at first appear to be immoral are more properly called tragic when the effects of scarcity are understood. For example, Walsh asks us to consider the case of a physician who has failed to provide a patient with an essential remedy.[14] Initially, we may be morally incensed. But then we are told that both physician and patient were at sea in a boat that lacked the necessary medical supplies. Or perhaps we learn that the medical treatment had just been developed and the physician had not yet been informed of it. On hearing the additional information, we are more likely to say "How tragic!" rather than to place blame.

Of course, we could carry Walsh's example a step further and ask why the doctor had failed to stock the boat with medical supplies or why he or she had not read the latest medical journals in which the treatment was described. But such questions might serve only to strengthen Walsh's point; for we might have uncovered a more general problem of scarcity. The scarcities that led to the tragedy might have been the physician's lack of time, energy, or memory. For example, the time that could have been spent reading about the new remedy might have been used to save the life of another patient. The more thoroughly we examine the effects of scarcity, the more likely it is that we will exchange the ascription of immorality for the appraisal of tragedy.

If the general conditions of scarcity tend, at times, to vitiate our attributions of moral responsibility, the same would seem *a fortiori* true of the conditions of dire scarcity associated with triage. And, in fact, some have concluded that *no* moral principles (let alone principles of distributive justice) are applicable in triage situations. For example, Dr. Jane Hunt, a psychologist and a participant in a conference on intensive medical care for newborn infants, gave this response to a discussion of the allocation of scarce life-saving resources: "I maintain (neonatal triage) turns out *not* to be a proper ethical question because there is *no* ethical solution."[15] Hunt argued that principles based on the "common good" and those based on the "special interest" of individual newborns could not be entirely separated. Thus, in her view, one approach is no more morally satisfactory than another.

If Hunt were right and there were no *moral* principles that apply in triage situations, then, of course, the narrower question of whether or not there are appropriate principles of distributive justice for triage would be misguided and should be abandoned. Moreover, even if one should argue successfully that some approaches to triage are morally better than others, it would not follow that these approaches should be described as just or fair (unless justice is equated with all morality, which is not the usage adopted in the present discussion). And, at least for the more limited argument that there are no principles of distributive justice that are applicable under triage conditions, one may find support in the writings of some moral philosophers. At least two different forms of the argument can be distinguished. I propose to examine both by letting David Hume represent one form and Gregory Vlastos the other.

Hume's Argument.

David Hume's statements concerning the conditions of justice remain influential.[16] According to Hume, among those circumstances in which a society would find principles of justice to be useless or inappropriate are: (1) a society blessed with a profuse abundance of every good thing, (2) a society in which every member is concerned with seeking the happiness of others as much as his/her own happiness, and (3) a society beset by extreme scarcities of even the most basic necessities. We can better understand what Hume says about scarcity and justice if we first look more carefully at the other two conditions that he says negate justice.

Hume begins by asking his readers to imagine a society in which "every individual finds himself fully provided with whatever his most voracious appetites can want, or luxurious imagination wish or desire."[17] Imagine further, Hume asks, that such a happy state of affairs requires no diligence, and life is simply an endless round of leisurely activities. Under such conditions, he argues, "the cautious, jealous virtue of justice would never once have been dreamed of."[18] After all, why should anyone be concerned with the just apportionment of goods when everyone already has more than can possibly be used? Witness the fact that societies usually do not establish rights of property or usage for abundant resources such as air and water. Only in those places where such resources are scarce do people concern themselves with questions of justice.

Next, Hume portrays an imaginary society populated by saintly beings endowed with completely generous dispositions. Such beings would be at least as interested in seeking the good of others as pursuing their own good. They also would be willing to sacrifice their own good for the sake of others, at least to the point where the harm accruing to them would be equal to the benefit thereby obtained for the others. Beyond this point they could assume that their fellow saints would be unwilling to allow more sacrifice. Such a society would be like one blissful family, completely united with mutual bonds of friendship and benevolence. Questions of justice, again, would be pointless.

Hume's reason for introducing these imaginary scenes is obvious. Human societies, as we know them, are neither blessed with superabundance nor peopled with saints. Rather, such societies are marked by moderate scarcity of many desired resources *and* some degree of competition for those resources.[19] These conditions of moderate scarcity and a degree of self-interest make the virtue of justice essential to the well-being of society. But, as Hume sees it, there are limits to the level of scarcity that a society can endure and still be served by justice.

Once again, Hume asks us to picture an imaginary society, this one faced with extreme scarcities. In his words: "Suppose a society to fall into such want of all common necessaries, that the utmost frugality and industry cannot preserve the greater number from perishing, and the whole from extreme misery."[20] Under such conditions, Hume contends, the laws of justice would give way to the demands of self-preservation. The underlying reason for this position is clearly revealed when Hume writes: "[W]here the society is ready to perish from extreme necessity, no greater evil can be dreaded from violence and injustice; and every man may now provide for himself by all the means which prudence can dictate or humanity permit."[21]

For Hume, the rules of justice are legitimate in so far as they serve the good of society. His concept of justice is closely linked to that of private property. Because of the conditions of moderate scarcity and self-interest, "civil society" requires rules governing the possession, utilization, and transfer of property. Indeed, these *are* the rules of justice. And their sole justification is their usefulness to the society. Thus, if society itself is threatened with demise due to dire scarcities, then all such rules of justice become otiose.

Hume is often linked with the later utilitarians.[22] And, in the broad sense of the term, his theory of justice is utilitarian. The rules of justice are chosen because of their usefulness to the society. He writes:

> A single act of justice is frequently contrary to *public interest*; and were it to stand alone, without being follow'd by other acts, may, in itself, be very prejudicial to society. . . . But however single acts of justice may be contrary, either to public or private interest, 'tis certain, that the whole plan or scheme is highly conducive or indeed absolutely requisite, both to the support of society, and the well-being of every individual.[23]

This is clearly some brand of rule utilitarianism. It is important to note, however, that Hume's justification for the rules of justice is not utilitarian in the sense that the term came to have after Bentham and Mill. Nowhere does he rest his case on the notion of the "greatest good of the greatest number." Rather, for the good of the *entire* society, as Hume sees it, there must be rules of justice. These are the rules governing property rights. (Interestingly, he follows the passage just quoted by saying: "Property must be stable, and must be fix'd by general rules.")[24] Such rules are not chosen because they are conducive to some happiness for the majority or much happiness for a minority. They are chosen and observed because the whole society needs them. As Rawls has argued: "[A]ll Hume seems to mean by utility is the general interests and necessities of society."[25]

In Hume's view, dire scarcities make void the rules of justice because the common good no longer can be served by such rules. If the majority cannot be kept from perishing and the rest must live in misery, rules of justice governing property rights would be inappropriate. Such rules no longer have utility in the broad sense of the word.

It is helpful to consider the illustrations that Hume uses to clarify his position. What purpose would be served, he wonders, in attempting to preserve property rights after a shipwreck? Would not the victims be justified in seizing whatever goods remained in an attempt to preserve their own lives? Or, to take another of his illustrations, if a city were besieged, would it not be permissible for the starving citizens to expropriate supplies of food? Hume's question concerning famine reveals his understanding of justice more clearly: "Would an equal partition of bread in a famine, though effected by power and even violence, be regarded as criminal or injurious?"[26]

With this question, Hume implies that an equal division of the resources would be morally justified under the exceptional conditions of extreme scarcity. But he does not consider the equal allocation of goods to be a principle of justice. Indeed, he emphatically rejects such a notion on the grounds that an attempt to achieve equality under the normal conditions of moderate scarcity would destroy the society.

Thus, at the heart of Hume's theory of justice is his conception of society and what is required for society's well-being. Hume places little stock in the contract theory of society. His arguments against Locke's version of the social contract are well known.[27] Hume sees society as having evolved through numerous forms of association and organization. The members of society have natural sympathy for one another, but they also have conflicting interests. Their sympathetic concerns are not strong enough to overcome the social tensions that tend to disorder society. For this reason, the "artificial virtues," including justice, must be taught and carefully maintained.[28] This is a gradual and painstaking process which is necessary if society is to survive.

In short, Hume conceives of society as a fragile association. It is held together not only by the natural sympathies of the members but also by the rules of justice that regulate property rights. He seems content to accept and preserve whatever distribution of property has already been established in the society. He cautions people to recognize their place in the social hierarchy and to be satisfied with that place. His greatest fear seems to be for the breakdown of society—a fear that is allayed by the strength of the rules governing the protection of property rights. These rights and thus the endurance of the social bonds may be destroyed by dire scarcities. When the granary doors are opened to provide equally for the starving in time of famine, society has collapsed and the rules of justice not only have been broken but have become purposeless.

Let us assume, for the time being, that Hume's analysis of the conditions of justice is substantially correct. If Hume's arguments are accepted, is it appropriate to speak of principles of justice for medical triage? Or do the dire scarcities of triage situations render the principles of justice useless? In order to pursue these questions, let us consider the two prismatic cases from chapter 2 in the light of Hume's doctrine.

In the case of the artificial heart, it seems that Hume's arguments do not apply. By our definition, the kind of scarcity anticipated after the development of a successful artificial heart would be called "dire." However, it would not be the kind of scarcity that Hume thinks negates the rules of justice. The scarcity would not endanger the lives of the "greater number," nor would it reduce the remainder of society to "extreme misery." In short, no matter how tragic it might seem, such a scarcity would not threaten to destroy the order of society, and there would be no point in attempting to confiscate the supply of artificial hearts for the purposes of equal distribution.

It is far more likely that the kinds of scarcities that might imperil the social order and threaten established property rights would be encountered in our other case, the earthquake. Even though the lives of the majority of the populace probably would not be lost, it seems certain that most of the city's residents would experience "extreme misery," at least for a while. The ability to preserve order following such a major disaster is a serious concern to those who are in charge of San Francisco's contingency planning.

The probability of maintaining order under the conditions of dire scarcity and the likelihood of people reacting in ways that go beyond self-interest are subjects for sciences such as sociology and psychology to explore.[29] As such, they are beyond the scope of the present discussion. But it is certainly not farfetched to think that the rules of justice, as defined by Hume, would be lost in the chaos following a major disaster. For example, the contingency planners for the San Francisco earthquake do not hesitate to include in their plans the expropriation of needed medical resources. Privately owned ambulances, drugs and other medical supplies, and the services of medical personnel would be used without concern for the normal patterns of exchange.[30] If one accepts Hume's account of justice as the preservation of the customary rights of others, especially property rights, then to a large extent justice probably would become impossible following a disaster such as a major earthquake.

It can hardly be denied that justice requires some degree of order. On this point, Hume is certainly correct. If dire scarcities reduce a society to the chaotic state of the war of everyone against everyone else, justice would be impossible. But if justice becomes impossible because of disorder, then triage also would become impossible. Both triage and justice depend on a modicum of order. The question, then, is not whether the dire scarcity of triage would make justice impossible, but whether the disorder caused by scarcity would make both triage and justice impossible. The answer to this question must be maybe.

Hume's close association of justice with property rights is problematic, as is evident in both of our prismatic cases. It might be argued, for instance, that the expropriation of a pharmacist's supplies, under normal conditions, should be called "unjust." But it is difficult to imagine *any* argument for calling such action unjust if the confiscation were necessary in order to save life during an emergency. And once the medical supplies had been so expropriated, the question would remain: If there are life-saving resources that cannot be given to all who are in need, is one form of allocaton more just than another? Hume's theory is not helpful in answering such questions about distribution. Indeed, with Hume's assumptions, such questions cannot be discussed under the rubric of justice.

The unhelpfulness of this position is also evident with the artificial heart. Who would be the "owner" of a successful TIAH if such a mechanism were developed? At present, the various working models usually carry the names of their chief designers or the institutions where they have been designed and tested. But much of the money for TIAH's development has come from taxpayers via federal government agencies. Even though some artificial heart development projects have been partially funded by private industry, the huge outlay of public funds would seem to point toward some kind of public claim on the technology. The implications of public financing for allocation of the devices, should they become clinically acceptable, is expressed by the Artificial Heart Assessment Panel in one of its recommendations: "Particularly in view of the substantial commitment of public funds for the development of the artificial heart, implantation should be broadly available, and availability should not be limited only to those able to pay."[31]

The assumption underlying this recommendation is that the benefits derived from publicly supported projects should be as widely available to the general public as possible. It might be an interesting thought experiment to consider what the moral obligations would be of a lone inventor who had developed and then manufactured a quantity of successful artificial hearts. But in today's interdependent societies, if ever an acceptable artificial heart is developed, it will not be solely because of the single-handed efforts of some isolated inventor.

Hume can hardly be blamed for developing a theory of justice that fails to consider governmental distribution of great benefits made possible by taxation. In the societies with which Hume was acquainted, such questions did not arise.[32] And yet, any theory of justice today that fails to include such considerations is bound to be judged inadequate.

We may conclude the discussion of Hume's position by saying that, however enlightening his statements on the conditions of justice may be, he has not shown that dire scarcities automatically render all principles of justice useless. We must grant the possibility that dire scarcities *might* lead to disorder, which would make justice impossible. On this point, there is no quarrel with Hume. But the problem with his position when applied to contemporary problems of distributive justice is his lack of concern for the distribution of goods to which no individual has exclusive property rights.

Vlastos's Argument.

There is another (and in some ways more troublesome) argument against the idea of finding any just solutions to the dilemmas of triage. Put simply, the line of reasoning is this: If a number of people have rights to a scarce resource and the scarcity makes it impossible to honor the rights of them all, then justice cannot be done. Somewhat different versions of this argument have been offered by a number of philosophers.

But because of its clarity, I shall take Gregory Vlastos's statement as exemplary.[33]

At the heart of Vlastos's egalitarian theory of justice is the following definition: "An action is *just* if, and only if, it is prescribed exclusively by regard for the rights of all whom it affects substantially."[34] (The term "substantially" is left deliberately vague, but it is apparently included in order to rule out the frivolous claims of those who would be only slightly affected by the action in question.) This concept of justice is based on the belief that, in terms of their intrinsic worth as human beings, all people are equal. This conviction leads Vlastos to argue that "one man's well-being is as valuable as any other's," and "one man's freedom is as valuable as any other's."[35] Thus, all people have equal welfare-rights and equal freedom-rights. But the most basic right, according to Vlastos, is the right of each person to have his or her other rights respected impartially.

The reason that Vlastos must deny the possibility of justice in situations of dire scarcity is already revealed in his definition of just action. An action can be just only, he contends, if it respects the rights of *all* who will be substantially affected. Thus, if someone's right to well-being, for example, cannot be fully honored, the action is not just. This does not mean, however, that the action is necessarily *un*just. It simply means that whatever else may be said about the action (for example, that it was loving, kind, courageous, and so on) the action cannot be called "just." Vlastos says: "When A helps one needy person, disregarding the claims of millions of others for the simple reason that he is in no position to help more than one out of all these millions," neither the words "just" nor "unjust" apply.[36] To use Vlastos's expression, such an action is "*non*-just."

Vlastos's position becomes clearer if we consider another of his illustrations and the observations he makes about it:

> Two strangers are in immediate danger of drowning off the dock on which I stand. I am the only one present, and the best I can do is to save one while the other drowns. Each has a right to my help, but I cannot give it to both. Hence regard for rights does not prescribe what I am to do, and neither "just" nor "unjust" will apply: I am not unjust to the one who drowns, nor just to the one I save.[37]

The scarce resource needed in this case is the life-saving ability of the person on the dock, an ability that presumably cannot be so divided as to aid both potential victims. In other words, Vlastos has presented us with a case of dire scarcity.

Just what the life-saving ability is (to throw the one and only life-preserver, to row a boat, to dive in and save one person) we are not told. It probably matters little, except that some forms of lifesaving could be more dangerous than others. According to Vlastos, the two drowning persons have a "right" to the help of the one on the dock. If we accept the well-established formula that the rights of one entail the duties of another,[38] then, in Vlastos's view, our would-be lifesaver has a duty to save both drowning persons. Since the two are "strangers" to the potential lifesaver, it is not entirely clear how he or she became so obligated. Indeed, others have used similar stories to show degrees of obligation depending on the former actions of the potential lifesaver.[39] Presumably, Vlastos bases the obligation on his already stated principle that everyone has an equal right to well-being.

Let us leave aside the difficulties posed by the presumption of the potential lifesaver's obligation, and accept Vlastos's assertion that the two who are drowning have a right to help. According to Vlastos, because both have such a right, because the right of only one can be honored, and because actions can be just only if they are prescribed by regard for the rights of *all* who are "substantially affected," no action in this case could be called "just." Nor could any action be called "unjust." To use Vlastos's language once again, any action in such a case would be "*non*-just."

It must be granted that Vlastos has not invented an idiosyncratic way of using the words "just" and "unjust." In one sense, his usage is in keeping with the poet's ancient formula that it is "just to give to each what is owed."[40] If both swimmers are "owed" the help of the rescuer, then in this sense of the term justice cannot be done. But Vlastos himself has stated a formal principle that provides the possibility of a different conclusion.

In the same essay, Vlastos says that his definition of justice entails one elementary right which, stated formally, is "the right to have one's other rights respected as impartially as those of any other interested party."[41] It is this imperative which Vlastos claims cannot be put into practice under the conditions of dire scarcity. But is this account of the matter correct? The answer obviously depends on what it means to have one's rights "respected impartially." If impartial respect means "equal satisfaction of desires" or "equal fulfillment of needs," then, by definition, dire scarcity makes such respect impossible. It is apparently this meaning that Vlastos has in mind.

But the right to have one's other rights respected impartially may be interpreted otherwise. This can be seen by reconsidering Vlastos's illustration. The two who are drowning, we are told, are *strangers* to the one who has happened upon the scene. Offhand, this may seem to be an unimportant detail, added only for spice. But, in fact, this element of the story is crucial; for we are led by implication to think of the observer as being *impartial*. The importance of this point can be understood better if we revise the illustration somewhat. Let us imagine that the rescuer notices that one of the hapless swimmers is calling for help in German, the other in English. The rescuer, we will say, understands both languages. S/he also hates all Germans. So s/he quickly throws the life preserver to the English-speaking swimmer, and smiles as s/he hears one last faint *"zu Hilfe!"*

This revised illustration makes the necessary point in a negative way. In this version, the rescuer could not be said to have *impartially* respected the rights of all who were substantially affected. Far from being *"non-*just," the action would be called, appropriately, "unjust." If, however, the lifesaver had overcome the hatred for Germans and had found some impartial way for deciding to whom the life preserver should have been thrown, it could be said that the rights of both swimmers had been impartially respected. Impartial respect, in this sense, would not mean honoring the rights of the swimmers by fulfilling their needs equally. Rather, it would mean *giving equal weight* to the rights of both swimmers. Equal consideration of the rights of both to well-being would certainly be more just than allowing prejudice to overrule the rights of one. Such equality of consideration would be in keeping with Vlastos's axiom that "one man's well-being is as valuable as any other's."

This same point can be illustrated further with a less bizarre example, this one involving scarce life-saving medical resources.[42] Each year about one thousand people in the United States are stricken with aplastic anemia, a disease in which the bone marrow stops producing essential elements of the blood including the white cells that fight infection. The majority of the victims die within a few months. Because the disease is sometimes associated with anticancer therapies, scientists at the National Cancer Institute (NCI) have been interested in studying it. To do this, NCI has constructed eight "laminar air flow rooms" which are near-sterile chambers. In these small rooms, the victims of aplastic anemia can live, free of the viruses and bacteria that otherwise would threaten their lives. But such treatment costs hundreds of dollars a day.

Questions about the propriety of patient selection for the costly therapy were raised because of a patient who has lived in one of the air flow rooms since 1972. The patient's father is a high official at NCI, and allegations were made that the father had used his position to gain his son's admission to the special program for aplastic anemia. According to the report, an investigation by a medical board at the National Institutes of Health led to the conclusion that the allegations were false.

Why was it necessary to conduct an inquiry to be certain that no impropriety had occurred? This case again reveals the point which needs to be made about the possibility of justice in triage situations. In the earlier case, the prejudiced rescuer failed the test of impartiality by not giving equal consideration to the rights of both swimmers. One swimmer was unfairly *excluded* from consideration. In the NCI case, questions were raised about whether a patient had been unfairly *included*. In both cases, impartiality of consideration, giving equal weight to the rights of all who are substantially affected, is the most basic question of justice. These cases teach us that, at the very least, some actions may be more just than others in situations of dire scarcity. Although we may not know what action would be most just, and although no action may be perfectly just, we are still able to discern which actions would be blatantly unjust. This conclusion may seem minimal, but it is hardly unimportant. As Edmond Cahn has argued, the sense of injustice gives an important clue to the shape justice should take.[43]

There is at least one more point that needs to be made concerning Vlastos's position. Once again his illustration of the unfortunate swimmers will serve us. Vlastos insists that the potential lifesaver's action can be neither just nor unjust regardless of which person is saved. But what if the lifesaver decides not to save either of the drowning swimmers? Let us suppose that the lifesaver agrees that s/he has a duty to save both swimmers. And let us add that it is a duty that can be performed with little risk or inconvenience to the potential lifesaver (for example, throwing a nearby life preserver).[44] Nevertheless, the one on the dock decides not to rescue either swimmer on the grounds that no just action is possible. Since the potential rescuer considers all possible actions to be nonjust, s/he simply chooses the most convenient nonjust action.

It is unlikely that Vlastos would agree to call the action of our imaginary nonlifesaver "non-just." And, in fairness to Vlastos, it must be said that his version of the illustration does not even hint at the possibility that the observer would not attempt to save either swimmer. Indeed, one principle of justice he enunciates would appear to rule out such failure to act. According to Vlastos, people have not only equal rights to the means of well-being but also, as a matter of justice, they are "entitled to this benefit at the highest level at which it may be secured." For the moment, let us leave aside the debate about whether such a principle is actually one of justice or should be more properly called a principle of beneficence.[45] The point is this: if justice demands the provision of the means of well-being at the highest possible level, then the decision not to throw a life preserver to one of the drowning swimmers would be unjust. Of course, Vlastos did not have this type of case in mind when he stated the principle. But if the principle can be applied to the distribution of "more or less," it would seem to apply with even greater force to the distribution of "all or nothing." Throwing the only life preserver would surely be a higher level of providing the means for well-being than leaving the life preserver on the dock. In terms of Vlastos's principle, it would be unjust not to throw the life preserver.

Even without Vlastos's ambitious principle, however, it is possible to speak of the injustice of not throwing the one life preserver. This can be done with a more modest principle which is not subject to the criticism that the distinction between beneficence and justice is being elided. The principle can be stated as follows: If a number of people have rights to a needed but scarce resource, the resource should be distributed as impartially as possible rather than wasted by being unused. The intuitive idea is that it is more just to provide a limited good to some people who have rights to it than it is to waste the good for fear that it cannot be provided to all who may have rights to it. This idea can be elucidated further by some comments G. E. M. Anscombe has made about a hypothetical case of medical triage.[46]

In the case discussed by Anscombe, the life of one patient is about to be saved by administering a massive dose of a particular drug, a dose so large that it would exhaust the available supply. Just then, five more patients arrive whose lives could be saved with much smaller doses of the same drug.[47] Anscombe argues that if the first patient is given the large dose, then none of the other five can claim that s/he was wronged. None can say that a portion of the drug was wrongfully denied him/her, because the drug had already been committed to the first patient. The main thrust of this argument is against the utilitarian principle, which would require us to pass by the first patient and attempt to satisfy the needs of as many patients as possible. But Anscombe also comments on the possibility of not using the drug at all:

> [A]ll can reproach me if I gave it [i.e., the drug] to none. It was there, ready to supply human need, and human need was not supplied. So any one of them can say: you ought to have used it to help us who needed it; and so all are wronged. But if it was used for someone, as much as he needed it to keep him alive, no one has any ground for accusing me of having wronged *himself*.[48]

Later, Anscombe adds the qualification that no one would be wronged by using the complete supply for the first patient "unless the preference signalizes some ignoble contempt."[49] With this proviso, Anscombe includes the requirement of impartiality. Thus, her analysis supports the principle stated above: scarce resources should not be wasted, but should be distributed impartially. Anscombe's version of impartiality seems to imply the use of a first-come, first-served method of distribution.[50] Whether or not this is the most appropriate way to avoid "ignoble contempt" will be discussed in the following chapters. For now, the important point is that wasting a scarce resource is an injustice to *all* who are substantially affected.

Summary

Dire scarcity—the lack of a life-sustaining resource that cannot be further divided and remain effective—presents difficult problems for any system of distributive justice. If the scarcity so disorders a society that both the consideration of claims and the administration of any rational plan of distribution become unattainable, then Hume is right, justice would be impossible. However, by definition, triage requires a measure of order and authority. And if the breakdown of society due to scarcity has made justice impossible, triage has also been made impossible. Of the two prismatic cases discussed in the last chapter, the kinds of scarcities (along with other factors) that would tend to render both justice and triage impossible are more likely to be encountered in the aftermath of a severe earthquake.

If there is sufficient order and authority for triage, then it cannot be convincingly argued that all forms of exercising that authority would be equally "non-just." It would be unjust to distribute the scarce resources in ways that did not give equal weight to the rights of all whose lives are in jeopardy. It also would be unjust to withhold a scarce resource and allow it to go unused. If dire scarcity calls for triage, and if triage is possible, then justice requires that triage *be* conducted and that it be conducted *impartially*.

This conclusion provides little in the way of substantive guidance. No specific directions for applying the general principles are given to the triage decision-maker. This is the work of the following chapters, as the substantive principles that have been or may be proposed for triage are examined. But in this chapter we have at least arrived at the conclusion that the conditions of dire scarcity do not necessarily render all principles of justice useless.

IV Principles for Triage: The Utilitarian Alternatives

From Formal to Substantive Principles

Offhand, the principle of impartiality discussed in the preceding chapter may appear to require the granting of completely equal opportunity to all who *need* the scarce resources. But such is not the case. As a formal principle of justice, impartiality does not prescribe the morally relevant criteria (such as needs, or merits, or utility) to be considered in deciding which persons should be included in the group deserving impartial treatment.[1] In other words, the principle of impartiality only directs the triage decision-maker to apply evenhandedly whatever rules are deemed "rights-establishing."[2]

This principle of treating equals equally is compatible with a multitude of substantive moral principles, including not only egalitarian but also utilitarian principles of distributive justice.[3] Indeed, the more important statements of utilitarianism have generally espoused the principle of impartiality. For example, Mill argues that it is "inconsistent with justice to be *partial*—to show favor or preference to one person over another in matters to which favor and preference do not properly apply."[4]

But the fact that impartiality is consonant with various systems of distribution, even those that appear to be in opposition, should not cause us to minimize the importance of the principle. Impartiality guarantees the regularity and consistency essential to the application of any and all substantive principles of justice. Despite the fact that it cannot serve as the final arbiter for competing substantive principles, it is an im-

60

portant first step in establishing a just course of action for the triage decision-maker.

It is the work of this chapter to go beyond the principle of impartiality and to begin an examination of substantive and procedural principles for triage. For the most part, these principles have actually been used or proposed for triage situations or in contexts that may be considered somewhat analogous, such as the oft-discussed lifeboat situations. In many respects, the list of principles discussed in this chapter and the following chapter resembles a recital of the philosophers' perennial quest for *the* right principle on which to establish a system of distributive justice. In summarizing the traditional "canons of distributive justice," Rescher includes the following: "equality, need, ability, effort, productivity, public utility, and supply and demand."[5] Our question is whether or not one or more similar "canons" can appropriately serve as a basis for establishing rights to medical resources under the conditions of dire scarcity. In order to facilitate a discussion of the proposed principles, they will be examined in the light of the prismatic cases described in chapter 2. An important test for any principle of justice consists of thought experiments in which the principle is "tried out" in the context of specific cases, either actual or hypothetical.

Before turning to the various alternatives, however, it is necessary to discuss briefly a view that may have the effect of thwarting the consideration of other principles. It is sometimes argued that triage is strictly a medical problem and consequently the selection of patients should be left entirely to the physician(s) in charge. As we saw in an earlier chapter, this view squares with what has been commonly practiced in the past. And it is not unusual for physicians to criticize any triage process that does not rely completely on the judgment of medical personnel.[6] The report of a conference of the American College of Cardiology is typical. A discussion of the "serious questions of distribution of scarce, life-saving resources" led to the conclusion that each decision must be made in light of the exigencies of the particular case in question. Consequently, it must be a "medical decision." The report indicates that physicians should become apprised of "ethical, social, economic, legal and theologic considerations," but then adds, "In the individual case situation, the decision is properly made by the responsible physician."[7]

Whether or not to "let the doctor decide" is a question of legitimacy of authority. If the decision-making power has been granted in harmony with right principles, then the authority is legitimate. But to confuse the question of *who* should decide with the question of *how* the decisions should be made would be an obvious mistake. Nevertheless, as Kass observes in discussing the distribution of scarce life-saving medical resources: "Problems of distributive justice are frequently mentioned and discussed, but they are hard to resolve in a rational manner. . . . The question of how to distribute often gets reduced to who shall decide how to distribute."[8]

One of the hazards of reducing the question of distribution to the question of authority is that the principles that actually govern the distribution will remain unexamined. For example, underlying the let-the-physician-decide approach *may* be a disguised appeal to another principle, "to each according to the probability of medical success." Since medical personnel are likely the most capable of making the necessary predictions, it would seem reasonable to leave the allocative decision to them. But the likelihood of a favorable medical outcome is but one possible criterion for triage decisions, one that will be discussed below and, it might be added, one that may be problematic from the perspective of distributive justice.

Whatever the merits of leaving all triage decisions to physicians, one thing is certain: the questions of distributive justice are not thereby nullified. Unless triage decisions are to be totally capricious, they must be based on *some* criteria, and these criteria can and should be scrutinized from the perspective of justice. Triage presents us not only with problems of medical skill but also with questions of human existence and human values. Regardless of who the decision-maker(s) may be, if a principled approach is sought, then one or more of the following principles is likely to come up for consideration.

In later chapters, more attention will be given to the underlying patterns of moral justification. But in order to facilitate that analysis the principles are arranged in the two basic categories that have emerged in earlier chapters: egalitarian principles and utilitarian principles. In one way or another the utilitarian principles represent "maximizing strategies" that aim to achieve the greatest amount of good (variously interpreted) or "minimizing strategies" that seek to reduce the amount of potential harm. The egalitarian principles, on the other hand, are generally viewed as attempts to maintain or restore the equality of the persons in need. The discussion moves first to a consideration of utilitarian principles.

Utilitarian Principles

U-1. Priority Given to Those for whom
Treatment Has the Highest Probability of
Medical Success

In accordance with this principle, candidates for scarce life-saving medical resources would be given priority if it appeared they had the best chances of deriving the most medical benefit from the treatment. Medical benefit in this case would be interpreted, of course, as significantly improved chances for some additional life. As seen in chapter 1, this has come to be the most commonly accepted approach to triage in military and disaster medicine, and it remains the dominant principle of triage planning for future disasters such as the next San Francisco earthquake. Under the principle, those who will probably live even without treatment and those who will probably die even if treated are left aside in order to treat first those who will probably live *only* if treated. The good to be maximized with this strategy, at least with the most obvious meaning of the principle, is the number of saved lives, and the harm to be minimized is the number of deaths. Let us refer to this as the medical success principle.

Use of the medical success principle is not limited to military and disaster medicine. In fact, if we consider the prismatic cases, it is easy to see how the principle could be applied more precisely in the case of a new medical technology such as TIAH. And, if experience allocating renal dialysis is any indication, some fairly elaborate attempts to assess the probability of medical success may be conducted. During the early years of renal dialysis, for example, some facilities went so far as to administer intelligence and personality tests in order to predict better the relative chances of successful treatment.[9] Both the very young and the very old were generally excluded from dialysis ostensibly because the probability of successful treatment was considered lower for them.[10]

The measure of prominence given to the medical success principle has, of course, varied among the thinkers who have reflected on the morality of triage. But, in one way or another, virtually all have recognized the legitimacy of the principle.[11] One of those who gives the medical success principle a place of considerable importance is Nicholas Rescher. "It is clear," he writes, "that the relative likelihood of success is a legitimate and appropriate factor in making a selection within the group of qualified patients."[12] Rescher argues that what he calls the "prospect-of-success factor" should weigh heavily at two points in the decision-making process: in a general way during the initial screening in order to pick a group of suitable candidates, and more particularly in the case-by-case comparison for the final selection of recipients. Another, similar statement is offered by Young: "In a situation of scarcity, priority should be given to treating those who fall within the category for which there is reliable evidence (antecedently available) of a markedly higher rate of successful treatment."[13]

The intuitive appeal of the medical success principle is strong. It would seem entirely irrational to waste a scarce resource on someone whose life could not thereby be saved while someone else whose life could be sustained by the resource goes without. But it would be a mistake to think that the principle is completely without problems. There are both conceptual and practical difficulties, which must be addressed if the principle's place in any scheme of triage is to be clearly understood.

One of the most obvious conceptual problems has to do with the multiple meanings of "success" in the context of triage. In order for it to be said that a person needs a particular medical resource, there must be some reasonable probability that the treatment will be at least minimally successful. In the case of triage, as it is understood here, this means that there must be a reasonable chance that the medical resource will at least prevent the harm of death. But after a number of patients have passed this minimal test of medical acceptability, it still may be possible to differentiate further their relative chances for medical success. This is so because in practice the initial assessment of medical need and the probability of medical success is likely to be focused rather narrowly on the patient's physical condition, especially the particular malady or injury. But the odds on medical success also may take into account many other factors such as the patient's willingness to follow instructions, will power, intelligence, and so forth. Moreover, the meaning of success may be expanded to include not only the immediate saving of life but also the *length* of life saved and the *quality* of that life. Indeed, if enough information were available, different odds for varying levels of success presumably could be established for each patient. Medical science has not progressed to the place where such exact and certain prognoses are generally possible. So Young's insistence that there be "reliable evidence (antecedently available) of a markedly higher rate of successful treatment" could hardly be understood like a law of physics, especially not in the case of a new medical therapy like TIAH during the early stages of its clinical use. But the inclusion and refinement of additional parameters undoubtedly would enhance the ability to make more accurate predictions of medical success and at the same time would permit a broadening of the definition of success.

It is at this point that two objections to the principle of medical success may be raised. If predictions of medical success are based in part on such factors as intelligence and will power, is there not a high probability that personal or social class biases will affect the predictions unfairly? And if the definition of success is broadened to include length of life and quality of life, is it not again likely that biases such as a prejudice against the elderly will affect the outcome?

Both of these criticisms have been made by those who have been especially concerned about respecting the basic equality of all the candidates in triage. For example, Sanders and Dukeminier write:

Social worth considerations, as well as unconscious biases, can secrete themselves within a medical or psychiatric evaluation. Hence selection procedures ought to be devised which keep these judgments as free as possible from such considerations.[14]

Ramsey echoes the same concern when he worries about "the social worth considerations hidden in many a medical and psychiatric judgment.[15]

People who share this concern are not likely to be comforted by the record of renal dialysis allocation during the days of its scarcity. In addition to the intelligence tests and psychiatric evaluations already mentioned, attempts to evaluate the probability of medical success included consideration of the emotional support of the patient's family, the patient's past record of reliability, and even the availability of transportation.[16] It hardly can be denied that such factors might affect the probability of successful treatment. But it is also easy to see how the same factors might serve as less than subtle measurements of social worth.

It should be noted that none of the authors just cited objects to the medical success principle per se. Ramsey, for example, assumes that the candidates in triage are "medically eligible." The concern is that medical evaluations will mask the impingement of other criteria, particularly judgments of social worth. Of course, if social worth considerations are deemed just, as they are by Rescher and Young, then the criticism that evaluations of the probability of medical success may actually be social worth evaluations in disguise has little force. But this is an issue that will be taken up later. For now, it should be sufficient to note that, in many instances, estimates of potential medical success may be very difficult to separate from social worth evaluations.

The problem of determining the meaning of medical success is not often mentioned in discussions of triage. In the writings both of those stressing the need to estimate probabilities of success and those cautioning about possible abuses, the meaning of "success" is often vague or ambiguous. For example, neither Rescher nor Young, both of whom use the expression, gives a definition. This lack of definition is not problematic if all that is meant by success is that the therapy will extend the patient's life for some indefinite period of time.

But it is clear that a quite different meaning is often implied. In his arguments for giving priority to patients with better chances of success, Rescher states: "It is on grounds of this sort that young children . . . are generally ruled out as candidates for haemodialysis.''[17] With this example, Rescher provides an illustration of some of the possible ambiguities in the concept of medical success. It is true that children were excluded from early dialysis programs partly because they were considered incapable of coping with the rigors of the treatment regimen. But there was also another reason: dialysis was thought to prevent the normal onset of puberty. As evidence mounted that dialysis could be conducted without serious harm to growth and development, centers moved toward accepting more children.[18] Clearly, the concern for ''success'' that led to the exclusion of children had much to do with predictions about the quality of their lives as well as the probability of preserving life itself. The same was probably true of the exclusion of people over fifty-five, although in the case of the elderly an additional concern about the *length* of the life being preserved also undoubtedly had some affect.

The inclusion of quality-of-life and length-of-life considerations in estimating the probability of medical success introduces two additional kinds of relative judgments. Concern is not just over the relative probability that the therapy will sustain life, but also over the probability that the life thus sustained will be of some relative length and at some relative quality. These additional success considerations greatly complicate the process of assessment, both technically and morally. It is difficult enough to weigh the various factors that may affect the life-saving efficacy of a medical treatment. And it may be seriously questioned whether human beings have the capacity to compare the worth of X years of life at A quality with Y years of life at B quality.

Consider two candidates needing one available TIAH. One patient is young and has diabetes. The other is over sixty-five but has no serious diseases other than heart disease. Questions of fairness aside for the moment, is there any calculus that would make possible a ranking of the value of these two lives? Adding more details to the example probably would serve only to complicate the comparison. It seems clear that the principle of medical success is least troublesome when interpreted as narrowly as possible to mean the probability of extending life itself. Whenever possible, judgments about whether or not a life-saving therapy is worth the trouble in light of the quality or length of life expected are best left to the one who knows most about the patient's overall life plan, namely, the patient.

One final criticism of the medical success principle (no matter how narrowly or broadly it is interpreted) deserves mention at this point. The argument is offered by Fried.[19] He denounces what he calls the "economic model" of health care delivery.[20] Such a model, he says, tends to favor the most salvageable patient or category of patients in the name of efficiency. At the heart of Fried's argument is the conviction that patients have certain basic rights *in* health care. One of these is the patient's right to be given the best possible individualized medical care, without regard for the general efficiency of the health care system. In Fried's words: "The physician who withholds care that is in his power to give because he judges it is wasteful to provide it to a particular person breaks faith with his patient."[21] Some inefficiency may be simply the necessary price of respecting the rights of the individual patient.

These rights, Fried believes, stem from a relationship of trust between the health care provider and the patient. Such rights are sufficiently strong that they may take precedence even over the requirement of equity. Fried grants that the "economic model" may be what is "dictated by the battlefield or emergency situation."[22] But, he says, one commits the "fallacy of the lowest common denominator" if practices deemed necessary in emergency situations are extended to the everyday delivery of health care. And he argues that the morally appropriate action in the ordinary practice of medicine is to treat patients according to their place in the queue.

The force of Fried's argument is probably most obvious if we consider the possibility of withdrawing life-saving resources from one patient in order to give them to another with a better prognosis. Such a practice would be morally offensive in all but the most extreme emergencies. And even then it would likely call forth feelings of profound regret from any morally sensitive person. But since Fried allows for the practice on the battlefield and in other emergencies, there is no quarrel about the emergency situation.

It is not difficult, however, to imagine numerous triage situations in which Fried's criticisms of the "economic model" would be less telling. For example, the selection of an artificial heart recipient might involve a number of physicians making a joint decision about which of several medically needy candidates should receive the device. Knowledge of the patients' needs and the initiation of medical care may both have predated the development of the artificial heart. Thus, organizing the candidates in a queue (how would it be formed?) would be of dubious worth. And in such a case, appealing to a relationship of trust between an individual physician and a patient would be inappropriate. It might be said that such cases should be governed by principles of justice that establish rights *to* health care and not rights *in* health care. But this distinction would be hard to maintain in practice. Medical care, especially for serious conditions, is more continual than the distinction implies. For the kind of situation Fried envisions (one doctor with one patient in the midst of medical care with other nonemergency patients waiting to be treated), his argument is convincing: people do have rights that ordinarily ought not to be abrogated in the name of efficiency. But there are numerous other kinds of situations in the practice of modern medicine where the medical success principle with its emphasis on efficiency may have a legitimate place.

In summary, the medical success principle is the standard approach in military and disaster medicine. It is, accordingly, the central element in the triage planning for the next San Francisco earthquake. The point is to save as many lives as possible. No ethicist known to have discussed the morality of triage has quarreled with the use of the principle in such emergency settings, although, it must be added, the principle is generally assumed and seldom argued for. The use of the principle other than on the battlefield or in time of disaster, however, has come under considerably closer ethical scrutiny. The broader the scope of factors taken into consideration in predicting success and the broader the definition of that success, the greater the concern on the part of some that the principle may contribute to unfair practices. The principle seems to be least troublesome when interpreted narrowly to mean the probability of sustaining *life* estimated on the basis of the patient's *physical* condition. But when interpreted in this manner, the principle comes very close to having the same effect as sorting patients on the basis of medical need. And, whether the interpretation is narrow or broad, the number of candidates who pass the test of probable medical success is likely to be greater than the amplitude of the available resources in many triage situations, including both of the prismatic cases. Thus, even if the medical success principle is given a place in triage, other principles also may be needed.

U-2. Priority Given to the Most Useful under the Immediate Circumstances

Under this principle, priority would be given to those candidates who could be of greatest immediate service to the larger group. Justification for the principle usually is given in terms of preserving the common good. But the common good, in this instance, is directly related to the immediate context in which triage is conducted and not to some larger, less related sense of social well-being. Thus, in the earthquake situation, for example, a nurse may be given preference over an entertainer not because the general social worth of nurses is judged greater than that of entertainers but because in the immediate circumstances nursing services would be more useful than entertainment. The nurse may be preferred, on this principle, in spite of the fact (and perhaps partly even because of the fact) that his or her medical needs may be less urgent. The point is to aid the recovery of those likely to be most useful as fast as possible either to prevent further damage (for example, from flood or fire) or to aid other victims. Let us call this the principle of immediate usefulness.

In his discussion of the morality of triage for mass casualties, O'Donnell contends that preserving the common good is more important than preserving individual good.[23] Drawing on a long tradition of moral theology, O'Donnell claims that the priority of the common good is required by "well-ordered charity."[24] This reasoning leads O'Donnell to the conclusion that "those patients whose immediate therapy offers most hope for the conservation of the common good should receive first priority."[25] Among his examples of people whose services might be especially important in triage situations, he lists government leaders, military officers and medical personnel.

He adds the proviso that each one in the favored group should have ''a positive and hopeful prognosis.''[26]

This principle of immediate usefulness should not be confused with the principle of general worth discussed below. The evaluation of usefulness O'Donnell has in mind is not based on some hoped-for contribution to the general good of society at some indefinite time in the future. Rather, the preference is given in light of immediate specific needs. This distinction will become more important as the discussion proceeds.

The type of triage situation O'Donnell has in mind, a disaster caused by nuclear attack, is similar in many ways to the anticipated San Francisco earthquake. And thinking similar to O'Donnell's is incorporated in San Francisco's current triage planning. Favoring those with special skills, it is hoped, will increase the available services for other casualties. And it seems feasible that such a practice could help to minimize the harm.

But it is far less apparent how the principle of immediate usefulness might be applied in the distribution of resources like the artificial heart. In this type of triage situation, it is difficult to imagine how any special skills of the selectees could be used to minimize the harm or increase the survival chances for those not chosen. Even if one of the candidates were a leading cardiologist, he or she could probably do little to improve the probability of continued life for the others. The need would likely be for more artificial hearts, not more cardiologists. An exception might be the case of a scientist on the verge of some discovery or development that would greatly improve the therapy for all patients needing artificial hearts. But this example is obviously unlikely. Any breakthrough the scientist might make would almost certainly take longer to become clinically useful than most potential recipients could afford to wait. Of course, it could be argued that selection of the scientist might benefit sufferers of heart disease as a class. But this is small compensation for those not chosen, especially when the stake is life and any direct benefits are likely to come too late to save the lives of those currently in jeopardy.

A more likely case may be imagined. Suppose that the scarcity of TIAHs is the result of inadequate funding and one of the medically needy candidates happens to be wealthy. The rich candidate promises to pay for additional devices and medical care if he or she is selected to receive the one presently available TIAH. Let us imagine, as well, that the lag time for production of the devices is not a major problem. In this case, would not the rich person qualify as having the sort of immediate usefulness called for by the principle?

This case may not be particularly farfetched. It will be remembered that just such a contingency was discussed by the Admissions and Policy Committee at Seattle's Swedish Hospital.[27] The attorney on the committee argued that they should be willing to accept a patient from outside the state of Washington if such a person were willing to finance the treatment of others. But the committee rejected the idea. Reports of the committee's work do not indicate the reasons for dismissing the idea, but it is probably safe to assume that at least one of the reasons was that the proposal was considered unfair.

The relationship of the concept of fairness to the various principles for triage, including the principle of immediate usefulness, is discussed in chapter 6. But is must be said at this point that intuitively something about the idea of favoring a wealthy person in the allocation of TIAH seems far more troublesome from the perspective of fairness than does giving priority to, say, a nurse in disaster triage. The differences in the two situations are too numerous to count. But the question is, are any of the differences morally relevant? For example, is the difference in moral intuitions attributable to the difference between emergency medicine and more routine medicine? If so, what is it that makes the emergency situation different? Or is it that the nurse in this case uses skills more dependent on his or her personal well-being than would be the case for the wealthy TIAH recipient? Or is the negative reaction to giving preference to the rich candidate actually a judgment of unfairness about the larger organization of a society that makes it possible for some people to buy more health care, especially life-saving health care? The answers to these questions are not immediately obvious. It may be that the moral difference between the two cases is more apparent than real. But this is a decision that is postponed for now.

To sum up, as with the medical success principle, the principle of immediate usefulness appears to face fewer challenges in an emergency setting such as a military campaign or a disaster than in the allocation of a scarce new medical technology. In military and disaster triage, the reasons for favoring a casualty with special skills—reasons such as preserving the fighting strength or increasing the number of available medical personnel—seem clearly justified in terms of serving the common good. But in triage for new medical technologies the reasons for favoring a candidate with special skills seem vague. Indeed, it is difficult even to imagine realistic occasions in which the principle could be applied to the allocation of a resource like TIAH. Giving priority to a wealthy benefactor of other medically needy patients is perhaps the least farfetched possibility. But, at least on first view, such an application seems unfair.

U-3. Priority Given to Those Who Require Proportionately Smaller Amounts of the Resources

Let us call this the principle of conservation. For an example of this approach, we may refer once again to an imaginary case invented by Foot:

> We are about to give a patient who needs it to save his life a massive dose of a certain drug in short supply. There arrive, however, five other patients each of whom could be saved by one-fifth of that dose. We say with regret that we cannot spare our whole supply of the drug for a single patient. . . . We feel bound to let one man die rather than many if that is our only choice.[28]

Why should we feel so ''bound''? Foot's answer is clear: If we do not have the resources to save all the patients, then, so long as we do not *intend* the death of any, we should divide the scarce resources so as to save the greatest possible number of lives.

The principle of conservation suggests maximizing strategies which could be better applied in military and disaster medicine. Resources such as plasma, drugs, and the time of medical personnel could be allocated in ways intended to maximize efficiency. By hypothesis, the scarcity would be dire because not all lives could be saved given the available resources. But, by using the resources for those who would need proportionately less, more lives might be saved.

Potential use of the principle in the case of the artificial heart is less apparent. This is so primarily because of the indivisibility of the scarce resource in question. Several candidates cannot share one artificial heart. It is not difficult, however, to imagine other therapies in which the conservation principle would be applicable. (For example, the principle was very important in the first clinical use of penicillin.) And even with TIAH some applications might be made. The patient might be excluded, for instance, if his or her condition would require a disproportionate amount of the medical personnel's time, or if predicted complications could create a financial burden ultimately resulting in an inability to help other patients.

The basic idea of the conservation principle, then, is simple enough: allocate the scarce resources in such a way as to save as many lives as possible. But further clarification is necessary. Consider, for example, the version of the principle offered by Young: "Other things being equal, preference will [should?] be given to those candidates who will not require a disproportionate share of the available scarce resources."[29]

The most obvious term needing analysis is "disproportionate." It cannot mean simply that one patient is likely to require somewhat more of the resources. To illustrate, if there were only two candidates and the available resources were sufficient to save the life of either one but not both, then in terms of saving more lives there would be no greater efficiency to be gained from favoring the patient needing fewer resources. Disproportionate must mean, then, that the resources saved by passing up one candidate (or group of candidates) are sufficient to keep alive at least two other candidates (or another group of candidates greater by at least one person). Put more simply, there must be adequate reason to think that application of the conservation principle will result in the preservation of at least one additional life.

The need for further clarification appears again if we ask the following question: Must the saving of at least one additional life be the life of someone whose needs are already known? In other words, when it is decided that a patient would require a disproportionate amount of the resources, must it be obvious that there are at least two others whose lives are currently in jeopardy for lack of the resource? Or may the principle of conservation be applied with an eye toward the anticipated needs of future candidates? Take the case of a patient brought to an emergency room with internal bleeding. During the treatment, which includes numerous blood transfusions, it is observed that the patient may exhaust the readily available supply of whole blood. Does the conservation principle call for a decision to set some limit on the number of transfusions because of the likelihood that at least two other patients may require life-saving transfusions before the supply can be replenished?

It seems clear that the conservation principle is least problematic when applied to a group of patients whose needs have arisen more or less simultaneously. But even so, there is still a major moral objection to the conservation principle that deserves mention. That objection may be illustrated by referring to a well-established doctrine of Anglo-American jurisprudence. In the case conceived by Foot, the physician who was on the verge of giving one patient a large dose of a scarce drug but stopped in order to treat five others would be legally guilty of the wrongdoing known technically as abandonment.[30] According to this doctrine, once a physician has begun to treat a patient, the physician cannot terminate the relationship without the patient's consent and without being certain that the patient has a reasonable opportunity to continue being adequately cared for by another physician. Even in the case of a disaster, it is not clear that the doctrine of abandonment is nullified.[31] Of course, legal liability in such cases would be very improbable, but in most states no provision is made for exceptions to the doctrine of abandonment in times of emergency.

The legal doctrine of abandonment reveals a moral concern for the preservation of trust relationships—a concern of the sort expressed earlier by Fried. As Fried sees it, a physician who leaves the care of one patient to take up the care of others for the sake of efficiency is like one who has broken a solemn promise. Faith has been broken. The patient's rights have been abrogated. Fried uses the example of renal dialysis: ''The physician would violate his obligation to his patient and the patient's right to the physician's fidelity, if he withheld dialysis on the ground that it is inefficient to devote these kinds of resources to this kind of patient."[32]

This argument is powerful. There is no question that there are moral grounds for considering abandonment prima facie wrong. But, as was seen to be the case when the same type of objection was raised in conjunction with the medical success principle, the criticism loses force if the triage decisions are being made about a group of patients whose needs have become apparent almost simultaneously and whose treatment with scarce resources has not yet begun. If any utilitarian principles are deemed morally appropriate in such cases (and it seems that some would be), then surely the principle of conservation would be among them. For Fried's objection to be cogent, there must be a situation in which a queue could be formed in some morally relevant way so that the claims of the patients at the front could be said to take precedence over the claims of those at the end of the line. The formation of a queue may establish legitimate expectations. And, without question, medical personnel establish a morally relevant relationship of trust once treatment of the patient has begun. But Fried himself recognizes that his principle of rights *in* health care may be overridden for the sake of efficiency in the emergency situation. He offers no criteria, however, for deciding when (or why) the emergency is pressing enough to justify departure from an otherwise valid principle. In this Fried is not alone. There is no lack of other authors who grant a similar exception but who fail to state clearly the exception-making criteria.

The principle of conservation joins the first two utilitarian principles in being more obviously applicable and less problematic in the emergency situation than in the allocation of some scarce new life-saving technology. The principle depends for its application on the ability to compare two or more distributive schemes and select the one likely to save at least one more life than any of the other alternatives. In the more routine practice of medicine the patient's right not to be abandoned may veto any application of the principle of conservation. But it is generally agreed that the emergency situation is an exception. Plausible reasons for this kind of exception, it is hoped, will become clear as the discussion proceeds.

U-4. Priority Given to Those Who Have the Largest Responsibilities to Dependents

This principle generally refers to the preferential treatment accorded to (or advocated for) parents. Rescher calls it the "family role factor," and he says: "Other things being anything like equal, the mother of minor children must take priority over the middle-aged bachelor."[33] In almost identical language, Young asserts: "[O]ther things being equal or indecisive a mother with young dependents ought to be given preference over a middle-aged spinster."[34] The difference being middle-aged makes is uncertain, but in the case of both statements not having children would clearly put a triage candidate at a disadvantage.

All the shorthand designations for this principle that come to mind seem somewhat awkward or even misleading. But for want of a better appellation, let us call this the parental role principle. As first stated, the principle need not refer only to parents or families. For example, the meaning of dependents could be interpreted more broadly, as Young does, to include those who rely on ministers or social workers. But, more often than not, discussions of this principle have focused attention on the special relationships of dependence within the family. Thus, for the sake of this discussion it will generally be more useful to think of these relationships.

It is not entirely clear that this principle deserves to be mentioned separately. It might be possible, depending on the kind of justification given, to subsume the principle under one of the others discussed above or below. Responsibility to dependents, for instance, might be fitted somewhat loosely under the principle of priority to those with greatest general needs. Thus, having a large number of dependent children might be thought of as one of the criteria of general neediness. Or if the good of the children is deemed paramount, the principle might be viewed as a means of protecting the most vulnerable. The principle also might be categorized as giving priority to those with a higher degree of general social worthiness. Thus, taking a broader definition of dependents, one might be justified in selecting the president of a nation over, say, a schoolteacher on the grounds that the president presumably has a greater number of "dependents." And if another human life depends on the survival of a candidate, as in the case of a mother with an unborn but presumably viable fetus, then favoring such a candidate might be thought of as satisfying the principle of immediate usefulness. Finally, just to show how diverse the possible justifications may be, responsibility to dependents may even be weighed in terms of probability of medical success. For example, one member of the Seattle Artificial Kidney Center's patient selection committee said that he favored patients with large families because "a lot of kids help keep a man from letting down, even when the going gets rough."[35]

It is not always possible to discern which of the above forms of justification, if any, is being offered. The authors who say that a triage candidate's relationship to dependents is an important consideration generally seem to assume that the reasons are obvious and need little or no exposition or defense. But even if it is left largely unstated, there does seem to be a dominant reason for this principle, a reason not among those just listed. It is the belief that a unique relationship between the candidate and his/her dependents should be preserved, particularly in order to meet the emotional, social, financial, and other needs of the dependents. In other words, this principle is aimed at maintaining the well-being of the dependents. Stated in utilitarian fashion, the principle would prescribe that triage lead to the greatest good for the greatest number of dependents. Of course, other utilitarian considerations, such as saving society the expense of providing for dependents, also may be deemed important. But seeking the good of dependents, especially children, appears to be the most important consideration in the arguments for the principle.

The parental role principle obviously would be of little use in the emergency situation following an earthquake. There would be no time to discover which casualties were responsible for dependents. Moreover, since the dominant concern is to save as many lives as possible, the principle almost certainly would be considered irrelevant. Of course, the concept of dependents might be broadened to include, say, those who rely on the mayor for leadership; it is not inconceivable that such a leader could be given priority. But should this happen, it is more likely that it would be justified in terms of the principle of immediate usefulness rather than in terms of favoring one whose ongoing relationship with dependents would be expected to meet a wide range of the dependents' needs over an indefinite period of time.

Giving priority to those heavily responsible for dependents would be more feasible and may also seem more appealing in the case of a scarce resource like the artificial heart. In most instances, it would be possible to ascertain a candidate's number of dependents and the relative degree to which they rely on the candidate. Among other things, financial factors could be weighed, and at least some attempt could be made to measure the impact of the candidate's death on the dependents.

But even if the needs of dependents could be calculated in such cases, would the parental role principle be morally justified in triage situations? When the stake is life, should the fact that one candidate has (more) children or the fact that one candidate's children have greater apparent needs bear *any* weight in the decision making? Philosophers have recognized both the importance of the institution of family for any system of distributive justice and the complications family structure brings to any distributional scheme.[36] It seems indisputable that family relationships create certain special moral responsibilities. But even if one family member is sometimes morally obligated (or at least permitted) to give certain types of preferential treatment to another family member, does this mean that family relationships are to be taken into account by someone acting in an official or quasi-official role as a triage decision maker? It must be admitted that this is a difficult problem. The philosophical discussions are inconclusive.[37] And the problem remains puzzling.

If we search for analogous situations in society which might give some clue as to ordinary moral judgment on the matter, the results remain equivocal. Special provision has sometimes been made for relationships of dependency, as federal income tax exemptions would indicate. But in some ways a closer analogy may be that of military conscription. For many years,special deferments were available to married men with children. Then in 1970, with the establishment of a lottery system for the draft, the deferment for fathers was eliminated.[38] The reasons for the change were no doubt manifold. (It was even claimed that the availability of such deferments encouraged hasty marriages and unwise procreation!) But unquestionably the most important, stated reason for terminating the deferments was the belief that favoring fathers was unfair. The fact remains, however, that for over two decades the fairness of a deferment for fathers was virtually unquestioned. And even in ending the deferment, special provision was made for cases of "extreme hardship."[39]

Draft deferments and triage practices obviously are separated by a wide gulf.[40] Perhaps there is little to be gained by the comparison except to point out that in both cases decisions of great moment to the parties involved have been affected by the fact of parenthood. In both instances, those with the role of parent have been given preferential treatment. In both, the primary rationale has been the good of the dependents. And, finally, in both situations critics have challenged the fairness of the practice and called for more egalitarian approaches such as a lottery.[41]

At this point, the question of the moral status of the parental role principle is left unresolved. It is sufficient for now to have raised the issue. It should be mentioned in summary, however, that the parental role principle differs from the first three utilitarian principles in at least three notable respects. First the principle is not concerned with efficiency in the ordinary sense. There is no attempt to "stretch" the available resources or favor particular candidates so as to save the greatest possible number of lives under the immediate circumstances. Second, compared to the first three principles, the family role principle is far more likely to be applied (or advocated) in a situation such as the distribution of artificial hearts rather than in disaster triage. Finally, and most significantly, the parental role principle shifts the reference of the "greatest number" for whom the greatest good is sought from the triage candidates themselves to a segment of the larger society, the candidates' dependents.

U-5. Priority Given to Those Believed to Have the Greatest General Social Worth

Without question, the one triage procedure that has stirred more controversy than any other is selection on the basis of general criteria of social worth. As described in chapter 1, this debate became particularly vigorous during the early years of renal dialysis. At that time, the patient selection process at many centers included an evaluation of the patient's overall worth to society. Decision makers, following this procedure, excluded certain kinds of patients such as prostitutes, drug peddlers, and prison inmates.[42] And estimates of social worth were also used as a basis for the *inclusion* of some patients. Thus, in some instances, the fact that a candidate was a church member, Scout leader, or Red Cross volunteer significantly enhanced his/her chances of being selected. Whether viewed as a means of inclusion or exclusion, the basic aim of this approach has been to seek the good of society by favoring those judged most valuable and disfavoring those judged least valuable (or most detrimental).

This principle, which we shall call the principle of general social value, would be all but impossible to apply in military or civilian emergency situations. It might be feasible to give priority to someone with specific skills needed at the moment, if those skills were known to exist. But this would be a far simpler determination. And it would be in keeping with the principle of immediate usefulness, which, it has already been argued, should be carefully distinguished from the principle of *general* social value.

Triage for TIAH, on the other hand, would obviously be different. More time would be available to ponder the candidates' "social worth profiles." Procedures could be established for making comparisons, complete with past records, letters of recommendation, and so forth. Moreover, with such an *expensive* and scarce resource, there would probably be a greater tendency to support the use of social worth criteria. Many people would probably find it "only fair" that the society that has paid for the development of a new technology like TIAH should make it available first to those who are most likely to make a good contribution to that society.

It is just this kind of argument that philosopher Rescher adduces in favor of the principle of general social worth. He contends that, in triage for some new technology, "society 'invests' a scarce resource in one person as against another and it is thus entitled to look to the probable prospective 'return' on its investment."[43] His rationale for this approach is clearly utilitarian. The triage decision maker should consider the interests of the larger society. In order to do this, Rescher recommends calculating the candidate's worth to the society by taking into account such factors as age, skill, past performance, and training.

Rescher recognizes that his proposal may go against the grain of an egalitarian society. There is reluctance, he knows, to attempt measurement of social worth, particularly when life is at stake. To illustrate this reluctance, he quotes another who says that it is impossible to select, say, a brilliant painter over an ordinary laborer. But Rescher asks: "What if it were not a brilliant painter but a brilliant surgeon or medical researcher that was at issue?"[44] The reason for changing the comparison from painter to surgeon or medical researcher is not made explicit. But given the context of the question it is obvious that Rescher believes the choice between a surgeon and a laborer would result in giving priority to the surgeon, unless there were other overriding considerations.

Rescher would not be surprised that it is precisely on this point that egalitarians balk. The principle of general social value is attacked on at least two levels. First, it is said that the principle is unworkable because there are simply too many imponderables in any attempt to calculate the social worth of an individual. Second, those who view triage from a more egalitarian perspective argue that even if the calculations could be made, measurements of social worth fail to give equal weight to each individual's right to life. Let us consider both of these criticisms further.

Childress gives a typical example of the first argument.[45] He reminds us that academic institutions have a difficult enough time trying to predict potential for scholastic success. But triage is certainly more complicated. People do not generally agree on what traits or talents should be most highly valued. And even if by some unlikely procedure agreement might be reached, there is no guarantee that similar valuations would be made again at some future time when new social needs and interests may have changed. For these and other reasons, Childress concludes: "We simply lack the capacity to predict very accurately the consequences which we then must evaluate. Our incapacity is never more evident than when we think in societal terms."[46]

Of course, a thoroughgoing utilitarian is likely to be undaunted by this type of criticism. If the problem of predicting net benefits to society is difficult, then why not develop more sophisticated methods of prediction? Joseph Fletcher, for example, suggests that in the future the complex process of patient selection may be "mathematicated" or "computerized."[47] In this way, many tangled factors such as cost-effectiveness could be sorted and given weight in calculating "optimific" decisions. This would be a scientific approach to the problem, says Fletcher, more like flying a plane with instruments rather than by the seat of the pilot's pants. And, it might be added, if our present ability to do such calculations lacks precision, this is hardly a reason to jettison the method. We only have to admit that the results permit a kind of rough, ordinal ranking, while we continue to evolve greater exactitude. If this method seems cold and impersonal, Fletcher reminds us that ethics is for the "tough-minded." Besides, he contends, it is a mistake to think of such utilitarian decisions as diminishing a high regard for the life of each individual. "It is not discounting the life of the individual, but balancing the interest of one individual against the interests of other *individuals*."[48]

But it is just this sort of contention that draws especially sharp criticism of the principle of general social value. This time the egalitarian objection is on a different level. For it is said that even if the principle of general social value could be made workable it would still be wrong on other grounds. In particular, the principle fails to recognize the elementary human equality that should accord, at the very least, an equal opportunity to life-sustaining resources. It is Fletcher's kind of "balancing" of the interest (the right?) of one against the interests of others which is of concern. If the person's general social value, however measured, counts in the balancing, human dignity, it is said, has been reduced to levels of performance in socially valued roles. Childress makes this point when he says: "The individual's personal and transcendent dignity, which on the utilitarian approach would be submerged in his social role and function, can be protected and witnessed to by a recognition of his equal right to be saved."[49]

A similar position against the principle of general social value is taken by Ramsey. "Granting that men are unequal in all sorts of respects," he writes, "these are not relevant moral features to be reckoned in deciding who lives and who dies."[50] Why not? Because, says Ramsey, the governing principle in such cases must be equality of worth as a human being.

To this point, our discussion of the social value principle has treated the principle almost exclusively as if it were concerned only with hoped-for benefits. That is, the principle has been viewed as giving priority because of a candidate's potential for doing some future good in society and not because of the candidate's past record of praiseworthy behavior. This approach to the discussion has been taken because most other treatments of the principle, whether attacks or defenses, also have viewed the principle in this way. Moreover, when the principle has been applied, as in the case of selection for renal dialysis, future potential appears to have been the main concern.

But, even though less prominent, the occasional treatment of the principle in terms of past performance deserves some analysis. It would be unwise, of course, to draw too large a distinction between social value as future potential and social value as past performance. It is hard to imagine measurements of future promise without *some* assessment of past performance. But when cast in the light of the candidate's good record, the principle may be based on a very different sort of moral justification. Rescher speaks of this difference.

As seen earlier, Rescher introduced the consideration of social worth in terms of the future good the society may expect from its "investment" of a scarce and valuable resource. He calls this the "potential future-contributions factor."[51] But Rescher also argues that persons who have benefited society by their good deeds of the past *deserve* special consideration.

Society, he contends, is obligated to reward people for past services. He calls this the "past services-rendered factor."[52] As Rescher sees it, such rewards are a moral obligation of society in keeping with the moral concept of equity. How should this moral obligation be weighed against giving priority on the basis of potential service? Rescher does not offer arguments, but in a footnote he says he thinks the two factors should be considered "on a par."[53]

Rescher realizes that this meritarian approach *may* be given justification in utilitarian terms; rewarding past services may, for example, prompt other people to render similar services and thus benefit society in the long run. But he believes that the utilitarian rationale is dispensable. The demands of equity alone are sufficient justification.

Without a utilitarian basis, discussion of the principle of general social value, with emphasis on past performance, would be inappropriate in the present section on utilitarian principles. But it is worthwhile, at this point, to attend to the possible ambiguity in the principle. Those who refer to general social worth do not always make it clear whether they mean former achievements or future prospects. But there is an important moral difference between *having worth* because of future promise and *being worthy* because of past services. As granted earlier, judgments of worth and worthiness may be integrally related. But they also may be viewed in opposition. For example, an older person may be deemed more worthy because of a long life of very good deeds. But a younger person may be seen as having greater worth because of the potential for many years of similarly good deeds. In terms of ethical theory, the "in order to" element of having worth is indicative of a teleological perspective. The "because of" posture of being worthy reveals a more deontological rationale.

To conclude, the principle of general social value, understood in its utilitarian, future-oriented sense, expands the reference of the "greatest number" for whom the greatest good is sought beyond the candidates themselves or their dependents to the society as a whole. Thus, like the parental role principle but unlike the first three utilitarian principles discussed above, the principle of general social value is not concerned with efficiency in the sense of attempting to save the most lives with the available resources. Again, like the fourth principle but unlike the first three, the principle of social value is more likely to be found appropriate in a situation like the distribution of artificial hearts than in the case of triage occasioned by a major disaster. In fact, the principle already has been widely applied in the allocation of one scarce new life-saving medical technology, renal dialysis. It has been defended by philosophers and others.[54] It has even been adopted by one government as a statement of national policy.[55] But the principle has also been the source of considerable philosophical and theological debate. Egalitarian challengers of the principle argue that determining a person's social worth is beyond human power both technically and morally. They contend that when life is at stake consideration of a person's potential benefit to society is a denial of human dignity and our basic sense of the equality of human rights. If triage must be conducted, it is argued, then the governing principles and procedures must be in keeping with the fundamental notion of human equality. It is to these proposed egalitarian alternatives that we now turn.

V Principles for Triage: The Egalitarian Alternatives

IN ONE WAY OR ANOTHER, the utilitarian principles discussed in the preceding chapter prescribe good-maximizing strategies. In other words, the goal is to achieve the highest possible amount of some appointed good (for example, the number of candidates' lives saved, the welfare of the candidates' dependents, the total happiness of society) as measured by the *aggregate* level of that good. The rightness of such strategies depends upon the sum total of the good produced.

As mentioned earlier, such utilitarian principles can be applied impartially and thus may be called "egalitarian" in the formal sense. Nevertheless, the utilitarian principles differ notably from the principles designated "egalitarian" in the present chapter. The following principles do not represent attempts to maximize the aggregate amount of any good. Rather, they call for the maintenance or restoration of equality for the persons in need. The relationship between needs and the idea of equality in such principles is strong. As Miller argues in his discussion of equality and needs: "[E]galitarians are committed to the view that justice consists (minimally) in a distribution of resources according to need, and . . . this forms a primary part of their conception of equality."[1] In various ways, the following principles build upon this basic conviction that the rights of people to have their needs met are essentially equal.

Lumping the principles into two categories, utilitarian and egalitarian, is not entirely adequate. Some principles do not fit exactly in either category, and others tend to overlap the categories. Nevertheless, the distinction between the utilitarian and egalitarian principles is fundamental. And problems with the classifications should not be permitted to obscure the differences that constitute a basic division of the proposed principles. These differences become particularly obvious as we consider the first of the egalitarian principles.

Egalitarian Principles

E-1. None Should be Saved if Not All Can Be Saved

Of all the principles that take human equality as a starting point, none can be called more egalitarian than this one. When not all candidates can be provided with some life-saving medical resource, the only way to treat them with absolute equality is to give the resources to none of them. The principle of saving no one is, of course, not properly a principle of triage at all. Rather, it is a rejection of triage; no one is selected, so no principles establishing priority are needed.

But one has only to think of the prismatic cases to realize that application of the principle of saving no one would be quite unthinkable in such triage situations. It would be preposterous, for example, to be confronted with a large number of earthquake casualties and decide to treat none of them on the grounds that there would not be enough time to treat all of them. Or if only a half-dozen artificial hearts were available for implantation, and even if 50,000 people needed the life-saving devices, it would be indefensible to refuse to save six people because the others could not also be saved at the same time. And there is little reason to worry that anyone in the medical profession would advocate such an approach. Ramsey is no doubt right when he says about the principle of saving no one that "the medical profession would not give the suggestion a moment's thought."[2]

Nor should they. Saving no one would wrong all of the candidates, even the ones who would not have been chosen under some selection scheme. As Anscombe puts it:

> [A]ll can reproach me if I gave it [i.e., a scarce life-saving drug] to none. It was there, ready to supply human need, and human need was not supplied. So any one of them can say: you ought to have used it to help us who needed it; and so all are wronged."[3]

But there is something about the principle of saving no one

that bids us wait and ponder. It cannot be denied that there is a substantial strand of Western moral thought that would prohibit the saving of ever so many lives at the expense of even one innocent life.[4] Moral philosophers have filled countless pages with discussions of trapped spelunkers, lifeboat occupants, and desert island castaways.[5] It may be worthwhile to consider one such discussion that sometimes comes up in treatments of triage, Edmond Cahn's commentary on the well-known case of seaman Holmes and the longboat of the *William Brown*.[6]

Holmes was convicted of manslaughter because he "jettisoned" fourteen male occupants of a leaky lifeboat in order to keep the boat from sinking. The judge in Holmes's trial told the jury that passengers must be saved before crew members unless the crew members were essential to the operation of the lifeboat. The judge also said that if decisions must be made about which passengers to save these decisions should be arrived at by casting lots.[7]

Cahn rejects this view. At the heart of his objection is the belief that some values are more important than life itself. He echoes the Talmud when he says, "Whoever saves one, saves the whole human race; whoever kills one, kills mankind."[8] Thus, Cahn denies the judge's solution of a lottery. In such a lottery, he says, there could be no "winners." All would have lost the essence of their humanity. "I am driven to conclude," he writes, "that . . . they must all wait and die together. For where all have become congeners, pure and simple, no one can save himself by killing another."[9]

Cahn's argument has undeniable force, and similar conclusions have often been reached by others. For example, in the celebrated British case, *Queen* v. *Dudley and Stephens*, the court found two British seamen guilty of the murder of their young sailing companion.[10] In a lifeboat and threatened with starvation following the sinking of their yacht, Dudley and Stephens killed a young man who was too weak to resist. By eating the young man's flesh, the two seamen were able to survive several more days until they were rescued. In his far-famed judgment of this case, Lord Coleridge, the Chief Justice, rejected the pleas of the defendants that they had been reduced to a state of nature where the laws of necessity prevail. The judge explicitly rejected the rationale for casting lots given in *Holmes*. Necessity would have been a legitimate defense if the murdered lad had been an aggressor. But the duty to preserve one's own life does not extend to the taking of other innocent lives. The judge recognized that Dudley and Stephens were under the most extreme temptation. But temptation is not an excuse for murder. Nevertheless, the judge allowed that if the judgment seemed too severe, it was the appropriate role of the sovereign, and not the court, to exercise mercy.[11]

Both of these oft-cited lifeboat cases represent situations of dire scarcity, in one case carrying capacity of the lifeboat and in the other food and water. But both differ from the conditions of medical triage in obvious and significant ways. Most important of the differences is the fact that in the lifeboat cases direct action was taken to kill some of the occupants so that others might live. Triage involves saving some and *leaving* others to die. The lifeboat cases would be more analogous, for example, if the scarce lifeboats were still on the sinking ship and decisions were being made by some presumably impartial person (say, a judge on shore who transmits instructions) about which persons to allow on the lifeboats. The impartial decision maker in such a revised version of the lifeboat cases differs in at least two significant ways from those who actually made the decisions. First, in *Holmes* the seamen who cast the male passengers overboard may be judged to have violated the special duties stemming from their role as sailors. The court's principal objection to the *Holmes* decision was *not* that only men were thrown overboard instead of some randomly selected group. Rather, the thrust of the judgment was against the crew, which saved its own members while casting out fourteen passengers. In his charge to the jury, the judge said that the obligation of sailors is to save the ship and its passengers even if it means sacrificing their own lives.[12]

A second important difference is that in both *Holmes* and *Dudley* the decisionmakers' own survival depended on the actions taken. But even if one should agree with Edmond Cahn or Lord Coleridge that no one is justified in saving his or her *own* life at the price of *taking* another person's life, this hardly means that an impartial decision maker is also bound to let all die rather than saving a part. To propose that none of the lifeboats be lowered because not all of the passengers can be saved is counterintuitive, to say the least. To paraphrase Anscombe, the lifeboats are there to save human life. If they are not used, then *all* who are in need are, in a sense, wronged.

But, in spite of this conclusion, something is learned from the classic lifeboat discussions, the courts' decisions, and advocacy such as Cahn's of the principle of saving no one. The spirit of any egalitarian principle is revealed in the deeply felt revulsion from choosing the sustenance of one innocent life at the expense of another. Underlying many a statement rejecting all criteria for medical triage is the belief that when life is at stake human beings should be accounted equal. This is illustrated by the official statement of the Government of Austria on the subject of providing people with a scarce and expensive medical treatment:

> It must be a primary objective of Governments to see to it
> that, in the sense of equality of human life, all individuals
> —irrespective of their financial situation—should be able
> to enjoy such a medical treatment. It cannot be accepted
> that selection is made among the persons who might be saved
> by the application of special techniques. It is held that there
> does not exist any criterion that could be applied for this pur-
> pose.[13]

But, however much one may agree with the egalitarian disposition of this statement, the trouble with such a view is that there are times when some life-saving treatments simply cannot be given to everyone. The first few doses of penicillin demonstrate the point. And the first few clinically successful TIAHs, when such become available, will represent a similar situation. An unwillingness to provide the scarce resources to anyone would almost certainly mean that they would never be more fully developed and improved so that they could be made available to all who need them.[14] Failure to state any criteria for triage decision making certainly does not insure an egalitarian approach. (Indeed, quite the opposite might be the result.) But if the principle of saving no one is deemed inappropriate, perhaps a more plausible egalitarian approach will emerge from the following principles.

E-2. Priority Given to the Medically Neediest

The Artificial Heart Assessment Panel, it will be remembered, recommended that patients be selected who have the "greatest need for implantation of the artificial heart and are suitable candidates." [15] The latter of these two criteria, medical suitability, was discussed above in conjunction with the principle of medical success (U-1). It is the first criterion, medical neediness, that is at the heart of the principle taken up now. Under this principle, the candidates with the most pressing medical needs would be treated first. We will call this the principle of medical neediness.

As stated earlier, the relationship between needs and egalitarian views of distribution is a strong one. Indeed, distribution on the basis of needs is generally understood to be the essence of an egalitarian approach to social justice. Miller makes this point in his discussion of a needs conception of distributive justice:

> [T]he principle of equality does not demand that each person should receive the same physical treatment, rather that each person should be treated in such a way that he achieves the same level of well-being as every other. . . . No serious egalitarian has thought otherwise. [16]

People have different needs. These needs must, therefore, be met in different ways if the same levels of well-being are to be enjoyed.

One who has attempted to apply such an egalitarian, needs-oriented, view of justice to medical care is Robert Veatch. Although his discussion does not deal extensively with scarce life-saving services, his position is nevertheless of interest. According to Veatch, "The health care program that is most just is the one that will recognize a claim to health care necessary to provide an opportunity, as far as possible, to a level of health equal to others'." [17] Veatch claims that such a system would meet the requirements of an egalitarian theory of justice—a theory he offers as an alternative to a utilitarian approach to health care. Ideally, says Veatch, health care would be distributed in such a way as to equalize *health*. This goal would, of course, have to be subject to the limitations of the current state of the medical art and patients' willingness to accept treatment. But at the core of Veatch's position is the aim of giving everyone an equal chance to be as healthy as everyone else.

One of the more obvious entailments of this theory of just health care is the priority given to those who are most ill. Veatch puts is bluntly: "We would target our efforts on the sickest."[18] At the macroallocation level, if choices must be made among various categories of diseases when it comes to funding for medical care, Veatch argues that priority should be given to those diseases that "constitute the greatest assault on one's health."[19] The thrust of Veatch's position is, thus, to give priority to that group he calls the "medically least well off."

This position is based on a premise that appears to have strong intuitive appeal: the most basic justification of a claim to medical care is medical need. In the words of Bernard Williams's well-known dictum (which Veatch quotes favorably): "[T]he proper ground of distribution of medical care is ill health: this is a necessary truth."[20]

Although Veatch is not primarily concerned with triage decision making,[21] his approach, favoring those with the greatest medical needs, is certainly not unknown in the development of triage in modern medicine. As shown in chapter 1, for example, Baron Larrey, who was probably the originator of casualty sorting in military medicine, gave priority to the most seriously wounded regardless of rank or other considerations. But, whether in triage or in the more routine delivery of health care, the principle of medical neediness must withstand a major objection: it is often likely to be very inefficient. Because efficiency is considered paramount, discussions of military and disaster medicine have generally rejected the approach of treating the most injured first. In the words of one of San Francisco's emergency planning officials, one must take the "hard approach" and "treat only those who are expected to survive if treated."[22]

In the case of allocating TIAH, the inefficiency of triage

based on medical neediness alone may not be so obvious. But it is not difficult to imagine cases in which treating the sickest would run counter to the principle of medical success.

Veatch recognizes the problem of inefficiency and attempts to deal with it. He admits that in a health care system that tries to equalize health by giving priority to the sickest "a group of the incurably sick who are the most ill must end up with *all* the medical resources," and the system will collapse.[23] But Veatch escapes this counterintuitive result of his egalitarian principle by suggesting that the neediest can only lay just claim to the resources if some good is likely to come from the treatment.[24] Later, he further qualifies the principle of medical neediness by arguing that the just claims to which medical needs give rise must be modified by other ethical claims, especially those of efficiency. On this view, the criteria that make health care delivery *just* are not necessarily the same as those that make it *right*. In adding this qualification, Veatch joins a number of other authors who argue that just claims to health care may be overridden sometimes for the sake of efficiency or aggregate utility, but who offer little or no help in establishing the exception-making criteria.

Can exception-making criteria be stated for those times when utilitarian concerns for efficiency should override claims based on medical needs? Is Veatch correct in suggesting that efficiency may be a right-making but not a just-making consideration? These questions continue to be at the center of attention in the present discussion. But what can be said at this point about the principle of medical neediness as a principle of triage is that it is at once indispensable and insufficient. To say that someone *needs* medical care means that some (further) harm can be prevented or diminished by the care. In the case of triage, the harm to be prevented is death. But once this basic need for death-preventing care has been ascertained, it seems doubtful that further gradations of neediness could be used to establish additional priorities among the candidates' claims. If greater medical need means that a greater harm can be prevented, then, in a triage situation, further gradations are meaningless. All of the candidates are faced with the harm of death. From this perspective, they are *all* needy in the strongest sense. If, however, greater medical need refers to being "sicker," say, in the sense of a more deteriorated physical status, then giving priority to the sickest may have to be balanced against the principle of medical success. And if greater medical need refers to need for larger amounts of the medical resources, then giving priority to those with greater needs could run counter to the principle of conservation. Thus, it is clear that the principle of medical neediness must be suplemented by other principles.

E-3. Priority Given to the Most Helpless or Generally Neediest

In the traditional lifeboat stories, when the ship is sinking and the lifeboats are about to be boarded, the customary words of the captain are "Women and children first!" Whether this scene is more from folklore than fact matters little; the *idea* has had an important place in common morality. The reasons for according such preferential treatment are complex and no doubt reflect a variety of social values. But if people were asked to justify the practice, one of the likely responses would be that those least able to fend for themselves should be helped first. Some version of the principle favoring the weakest, or the most helpless, or the generally neediest has had considerable moral influence. For example, Hans Jonas has offered the celebrated dictum: "Utter helplessness demands utter protection."[25] Jonas was not speaking specifically about triage decisions, but as the lifeboat stories demonstrate, this approach to distribution often has been deemed right in situations of dire scarcity.

It is difficult to be very precise about the notion of giving priority to the generally neediest or most helpless. This is so because of the complex array of factors that may cause a person to be incapable of fending for himself or herself. The condition of helplessness may include a wide variety of personal and social characteristics such as the lack of political power, social status, intelligence, or physical strength. And, of course, in a market economy one of the conditions most likely to affect access to scarce life-saving medical resources, at least in the case of new high technologies, is financial helplessness. The one feature that makes any or all of these conditions relevant to triage is the way in which access to life-saving medical resources may be diminished.

In the case of disaster triage, perhaps the most obvious application of the principle of general neediness would be to give priority to those casualties who are least able to care for their own physical needs. Included in this group probably would be young children, the elderly, and the physically or mentally handicapped. At the macroallocation level, it also might be possible to give priority to entire districts considered more helpless than others. Thus, for example, certain sections of a city might be designated to receive extra medical supplies or medical personnel.

The ways in which the principle of general neediness could be applied when the scarce resource is some new technology, such as TIAH, may be less obvious. Given the present structure of the health care system in the United States, however, one condition likely to jeopardize receiving such care is poverty. A somewhat ambiguous precedent for distributing scarce resources like TIAH on the basis of some general neediness such as poverty was set by the allocation practices in a number of renal dialysis facilities. But the use of such criteria was equivocal. In some cases, for example, people with greater financial resources were favored because of their ability to pay.[26] But, at least in some dialysis centers, indicators of financial well-being were studied in order to give priority to the poor. It was reported, for example, that the Miami Artificial Kidney Center gave preference to "indigents and those unable to afford treatment elsewhere."[27]

The question remains whether or not such centers would have given priority to the poor if those better off financially had been unable to obtain treatment elsewhere, that is, in a situation we have chosen to call dire scarcity. And, if so, it must be asked whether criteria of general neediness such as poverty are morally relevant considerations when making triage decisions.

In general terms, an egalitarian argument for a principle favoring the generally neediest would probably run something like this: Every person has an equal right to well-being (or happiness, or primary goods, and so on). Therefore, those who are most helpless should receive preferential treatment in an attempt to bring them as nearly as possible to a level of well-being equal to that enjoyed by others. Or, to borrow Vlastos's language, "one man's well-being is as valuable as any other's," so everyone has equal "welfare rights."[28] It might, thus, be argued that if health care resources are insufficient to meet the needs of all, then priority should be granted to the generally neediest.

But, whatever the strength of this line of reasoning with regard to the distribution of other goods, there are some obvious difficulties when applied to triage. When the scarce goods in question are the means to continue life, does it make sense to say that the generally neediest should be given priority in order to equalize their chances for well-being? Such reasoning would be less problematic if the distribution were not of the all-or-nothing type and if the scarce resources were not life-saving. In other words, the principle would be less problematic if providing equal *access* could be expected to result in something like equal levels of well-being. But, by definition, the dire scarcity of triage situations means that equal well-being is unconditionally impossible. Since life is the most fundamental of those goods required in order to partake of other goods, life and the means to sustain life are incommensurate to other goods.[29]

There is, however, another way of arguing the case for the principle of general neediness which may be considered more successful. The argument is based on the more general principle of compensatory justice. In this way, it could be contended that the generally better off have already enjoyed a good life. In giving priority to the generally neediest, even if it means allowing some of the better off to die, the balance of justice is being partially righted. If the generally neediest have been deprived of a decent life in the past, at least they can be given priority now in the allocation of life-saving medical resources. Some comments from another essay by Veatch illustrate the argument:

> At this point in history with our current record of discriminatory delivery of health services there is a special concern for restoring justice. Justice must also be compensatory. The health of those who have been discriminated against must be maintained and restored as a special priority.[30]

97

This line of reasoning probably would be most powerful if it could be shown that the least well off now needing life-saving health care were ill at least in part because of the past injustices which deprived them of certain social goods including adequate health care. The claims of compensatory justice may have considerable force in the routine delivery of health care that Veatch apparently has in mind. This is especially true if it can be demonstrated that the social system has contributed directly to the creation of a group of people who are not only the generally neediest but also the medically neediest. But compensation with health care that is both death-preventing and scarce would be difficult if not impossible to justify. Past social injustices often may be partially corrected by the various measures that have come to be known as affirmative action in such areas as school admissions and employment. But affirmative action in triage would generally seem strange and unwarranted. Few social injustices would be sufficient grounds for concluding that those who had reaped unfair benefits would thereby have lost their equal right to life.

The very nature of the principle of general neediness tends to make arrival at definite conclusions difficult at best. The lack of precision about the nature of the needs in question and the relation of those needs to just claims leaves the role of the principle in question. A decision about the justness of the principle is postponed until the last chapter.

E-4. Priority Given to Those Who Arrive First

This is the principle of "first come, first served," or as we shall call it, the principle of queuing. On this principle, patients needing scarce resources would be treated in the order of their arrival for treatment. If more candidates arrived than could possibly be given treatment, presumably some type of waiting list or queue would be established.

The principle of queuing could be applied in cases of triage. But application of the principle in the case of disaster triage would represent a departure from procedures that have become standard in modern medicine. For reasons that have already been discussed at length, queuing has never been the first principle of disaster or military triage. Only after triage has resulted in the classification of a group whose lives were likely to be saved if treated promptly might queuing within that group possibly be employed. Even then, other factors, such as a candidate's immediate usefulness, would ordinarily reverse the queue. In any event, arriving (or being found) first would seem to make little difference if scores of other casualties had needs that had arisen at roughly the same time.

Queuing for a scarce resource like TIAH is a more likely possibility. And a significant number of commentators advocate such an approach. Several practical considerations give queuing undeniable appeal. Patients would know almost immediately what their chances were of being selected.[31] If the odds looked unfavorable, they might seek treatment elsewhere. Moreover, the procedure of first come, first served has been the standard practice of physicians and hospitals in the day-to-day delivery of health care.[32] Finally, giving priority to those who come first has a simplicity that makes its utilization attractive. Other more complicated principles and formulas could simply be ignored.

In addition to these practical considerations, there are at least two distinct moral arguments in support of the practice of queuing. The first is that being at the head of the queue establishes a right to treatment based on the legitimate expectations of a relationship of trust.

In his argument for the "rightness of queuing," Charles Fried contends that human rights take precedence over more abstract social benefits.[33] Rights and their correlative obligations arise in the web of interpersonal relationships. When a health care provider encounters and agrees to treat a person seeking health care a relationship of trust is established. The provider must not forsake that trust either for the good of another patient who comes later or in order to maximize some good in the larger health care system. It is the responsibility of the provider to give *personal* care: to treat each person, one at a time, with the best available means to meet that person's individual needs. Fried concludes:

> So as far as the doctor is concerned, there is a queue for his services. And since it is better that some receive personal care

than that none do, and since he is in the relationship that he
is to those patients who are already before him, then he must
let those at the end of the queue take care of themselves.
True, it is not their fault that they are at the end of the queue;
but it is not the doctor's fault either.[34]

Fried's argument is most forceful in those situations when
an individual patient confronts an individual medical practitioner. Neither of the two triage cases we have been discussing
is likely to be of exactly that sort. Rather, a group of medical
care providers probably would be confronted more or less
simultaneously by a group of patients. Nevertheless, this does
not mean that it would be completely impossible to form a
queue, although of the two prismatic cases it obviously would
be easier in the case of allocating artificial hearts. The precedent set at many renal dialysis centers, which followed the
practice of first come, first served, reveals that the principle of
queuing not only has considerable support but also is capable
of implementation.[35] And it is just this practice that, Fried
argues, is most protective of individual rights and the concept
of personal care within a trust relationship.

There is another kind or moral argument that is also used to
support the principle of queuing. This line of reasoning is more
ostensibly egalitarian. The practice of first come, first served,
it is said, is in harmony with the basic principle of human
equality, or more specifically, equality of opportunity. Queuing is thus seen as a type of procedural justice in harmony with
human equality. The links between queuing, equality, and
justice are illustrated in a passage from Brunner:

> Let us assume that five persons have taken up their stand at
> the cloakroom counter side by side, and that a queue has
> formed behind each of these five persons. If the attendant
> were to proceed in such a way that, having served the leading
> person in one of the queues, she were then to serve the person
> behind him, who had moved into his place, and so on till that
> whole queue had been dealt with, before she as much as began
> to deal with the other four, the people standing in the other
> four queues would have every right to protest against unfair
> treatment. She proceeds justly by taking the leading person in
> each queue from right to left and from left to right. In this
> way everybody has to wait for the same length of
> time. . . . First come, first served; last come, last
> served. . . . Hence, justice is equality. Just treatment means
> the same treatment for all.[36]

We need not take time to quarrel with Brunner's simple equation of justice with the "same treatment" for all. (The context seems to indicate that he is referring to the formal principle of justice: treat equals equally.) Brunner's illustration shows how the principle of queuing is often viewed as a way of according equal treatment in terms of equality of opportunity.

The use of queuing also has been proposed as a means of assuring equality of opportunity in triage. For example, both Ramsey and Childress see queuing as a practical way to accord fair equality of opportunity to those needing a scarce medical treatment.[37] Ramsey mentions one hospital that, he says, affords "equality of opportunity by a policy of 'first come, first served.' "[38] And it is interesting to note that both Ramsey and Childress (and, for that matter, a number of others) consider queuing to be roughly equivalent to random selection by use of a lottery.[39]

The principle of queuing, then, in addition to having certain practical advantages, is backed by at least two different kinds of moral arguments: protecting the rights of persons in fiduciary relationships and according fair equality of opportunity.

There are, of course, a number of utilitarian criticisms of the principle. One of the more obvious is that the principle of queuing may run counter to the principle of medical success.[40] After the process of queuing has been in progress for some time, the persons coming to the head of the line will have been waiting the longest and may consequently be the least likely to benefit from the treatment. Ramsey, Childress, and others handle this objection by incorporating criteria of medical suitability in the queuing process.

E-5. Priority Given to Those Selected by Chance

This is the procedural principle of strictly random selection from among those potential recipients of a scarce medical resource. In one form or another, the procedure is a well-known way of deciding who receives some indivisible good to which more than one person have equally strong (or weak) claims. Whether by flipping coins, drawing straws, pulling names from a hat, or a host of other specific practices, the goal is the same: to leave the choice to chance. This decision-making method is not only familiar but also time-honored in many common situations (for example, which football team kicks off and which receives). But is a procedure associated with games and gambling appropriate for the allocation of life-saving medical services?

In the case of disaster triage, the answer is surely negative. But random selection for TIAH would be more feasible. And, indeed, just such an approach has been advocated by the Artificial Heart Assessment Panel. The panel's report states that if an initial screening results in a group of patients with roughly equal needs and medical suitability, then any further selection should be by some random method. Explicitly rejecting general social worth criteria and the ability to pay as ways of selecting patients, the panel wrote: "[W]e believe that random selection, as among equally necessitous patients, is a desirable principle."[41]

Evidence that such a method of random selection can actually be employed comes from the experience of some renal dialysis facilities. For example, it was reported that one Southern California medical center conducted an initial screening of the candidates and then left the final selection to chance. "The names of all needy candidates who pass this basic screening are put into a hat and drawn by lot until the program is full. The names of losers are retained for subsequent drawings."[42] It should be pointed out that the lottery in this example was used in conjunction with other criteria, including evaluations of social worth. The initial screening was used not only to determine medical need and suitability but also to rule out "alcoholics and criminals."[43] But there is obviously no reason that would make such social worth evaluations indispensable. And, in fact, other centers reportedly relied almost totally on random selection once medical need was established.[44]

The primary moral argument for random selection is that this approach best assures fair equality of opportunity. Potential recipients are treated with total impartiality. One candidate's right to life is given the same weight as any other's.

Or, in Childress' words, randomness "preserves a significant degree of *personal dignity* by providing *equality* of opportunity."[45]

There is also another type of moral argument in favor of random selection, one that occurs almost as frequently as the argument for equality of opportunity. It is often said that people are ill-equipped to decide who from among their fellow human beings shall live when not all can live. Leaving the choice to chance eliminates, so far as possible, human control of the outcome. This is the view that appears to be expressed in Paul Freund's oft-quoted statement: "The more nearly total is the estimate to be made of an individual, and the more nearly the consequence determines life and death, the more unfit the judgment becomes for human reckoning. . . . Randomness as a moral principle deserves serious study."[46] On this view, truer testimony to the dignity and worth of each individual's life is borne when human judgment about the relative value of it is kept to a minimum.

There are other points to be made in favor of the principle of random selection. Like the principle of queuing, random selection is relatively simple to apply. And although, in contrast to queuing, casting lots is not part of the routine practice of medicine, the randomizing process has become a familiar part of research medicine. The "randomized clinical trial" in which patients are selected at random for a particular therapy is now a standard procedure for the testing of many new drugs and medical treatments.[47] In the cases of both research medicine and triage, the process of randomization serves to eliminate the influence of certain factors considered to be extraneous.

Of course, triage situations supposedly differ from clinical trials in significant ways. Presumably, the life-saving efficacy of the scarce treatment would already have been sufficiently demonstrated so that it would no longer be considered "experimental." But such demonstration, it must be remembered, is always a matter of determining levels of probability. And since all individual medical interventions are experimental at some level of probability, random selection of candidates in triage could provide, as a "windfall," the opportunity for research if data were systematically collected and compared in an attempt to arrive at general conclusions. Indeed, just such a reason for random selection in triage has been suggested.[48] It is not our purpose here to enter the vexed discussion of what constitutes research, experimentation, and therapy.[49] Rather, the point is simply that randomizing patients for various kinds of therapy is not unknown to modern medicine and if utilized in triage might even be viewed by some as a potentially fruitful opportunity to conduct research.

But, in spite of the supporting arguments, both moral and pragmatic, many who have contemplated a lottery for triage have rejected the idea as morally repugnant. Perhaps the most often voiced objection is that selection by chance is an irresponsible abandonment of moral and rational decision-making. Put bluntly, random selection looks like an easy way out. This view was expressed by a surgeon and member of the Seattle Artificial Kidney Center's patient selection committee: "[A]t our committee's first meeting we seriously discussed selecting candidates by drawing straws. We were going to make it easy on ourselves by having a human lottery!"[50] But, as is well-known, the committee rejected this approach and chose instead to develop its own criteria for patient selection.

A more vigorous rejection of a "human lottery" is sometimes found among those who say that random selection is unfair. Failure, for example, to consider the candidates' potential social contributions or past record of meritorious action could lead to the selection of those who are least "deserving." Leach's comment about random selection is typical of this kind of criticism:

> Though this [that is, a lottery] would eliminate all subjective judgment [*sic*] values of "worth," it is nevertheless the most unfair system imaginable. To allow dice to choose between people would not only condemn some very "worthy" people at the expense of others; it would be a kind of treason against human compassion and responsibility.[51]

Thus, the lottery is often seen as antithetical to social worth evaluations. In a comment similar to Leach's, Shatin calls random selection "an extreme thesis for equality," which, he contends, would "reward socially disvalued qualities by giving their bearers the same special medical care opportunities as those received by the bearers of socially valued qualities."[52]

Finally, there is the objection made by Fried that random selection would be "unstable."[53] Fried cites TIAH as a case in point. He says that the general provision of artificial hearts to all who might need them is likely to be an "intolerable burden." Fried does not say exactly which method of allocation he would advocate if and when TIAH becomes available. But he rejects the idea of random selection:

> Nor is a lottery device for distributing a limited number of artificial hearts likely to be more stable or satisfactory. For there, too, would we forbid people to go outside the lottery? Would it be a crime to cross national boundaries with the intent of obtaining an artificial heart?[54]

Fried's objection is based on the difficulty of establishing and maintaining rational boundaries within which a lottery might take place. This is no small problem, and it will be explored in chapter 6. But, if territorial limits represent a problem for random selection, the same would seem true, to a greater or lesser extent, for most any principle of selection.

In summary, it can be said that the principle of random selection has generally been favored by those wanting to ensure equal opportunity. To the extent that these proponents equate random selection with queuing, it is because both are viewed as procedural principles capable of establishing equality of opportunity. What is more, advocates, on one hand, argue that triage by chance would eliminate, so far as possible, the need for fallible human judgments about the relative value of others' lives. Critics, on the other hand, see the use of a lottery as an escape from moral responsibility and, at least in the case of Fried, as an unstable and impracticable approach to triage.

The Possibility of Ranking Principles for Triage

It may be useful at this point to list in summary fashion the principles discussed in chapters 4 and 5:

Utilitarian Principles:

U-1. The principle of medical success. Priority given to those for whom treatment has the highest probability of medical success.

U-2.   The principle of immediate usefulness. Priority given to the most useful under the immediate circumstances.

U-3.   The principle of conservation. Priority given to those who require proportionately smaller amounts of the resources.

U-4.   The principle of parental role. Priority given to those who have the largest responsibilities to dependents.

U-5.   The principle of general social value. Priority given to those believed to have the greatest general social worth.

Egalitarian Principles:

E-1.   The princple of saving no one. Priority given to no one because none should be saved if not all can be saved.

E-2.   The principle of medical neediness. Priority given to the medically neediest.

E-3.   The principle of general neediness. Priority given to the most helpless or generally neediest.

E-4.   The principle of queuing. Priority given to those who arrive first.

E-5.   The principle of random selection. Priority given to those selected by chance.

It should be noted that the principles of both basic types are seldom mutually exclusive. Indeed, with the exception of the principle of saving no one, it is conceivable that all the principles could be combined in some elaborate decision-making matrix. Each principle could be given a certain weight and place in the order of application. Some of the principles might thus be used as means of exclusion. For example, if the odds on medical success were sufficiently low, the patient simply would not be included among these candidates from whom the final selection would be made. Other principles, such as general social value or general neediness, could be used either singly or in concert for making the final selection.

But there is an obvious queston which arises at this point: Is there any way to arrange the principles in some rank order that would be defensible from a moral point of view? Or, stated more specifically in terms of the present inquiry, is any ranking of the principles more *just* than another?

Perhaps the answer to this sort of question is negative. It is difficult enough to state tenable principles. Arranging them in some rank order may be considered overly ambitious. An example of one who apparently thinks so is Young. He lists five principles for distributing scarce medical resources and he also sets forth fifteen "suggestions" for implementation. But he makes no attempt to rank the principles. In fact, he says that "the principles have deliberately been left unordered *morally*."[55] Presumably, the triage decision maker who wishes guidance from Young's discussion must make do with an *ad hoc* balancing of the various principles.

If no further ordering of the principles is possible, then it is no doubt best to say so and relinquish any pretense of doing otherwise. But an explanation of the normative discussions of triage reveals a tendency to establish a kind of methodological presumption in favor of one or the other of the two basic types of principles we have outlined above.[56] These discussions generally incorporate a mixture of the principles listed above, both utilitarian and egalitarian. But these "mixtures" are generally weighted in the direction of either utility or equality. Either the prescribed approach is fundamentally utilitarian with equality on the basis of need introduced as a secondary consideration or it is fundamentally egalitarian with exceptions for utility or efficiency being made to bear the burden of proof.

For example, Young says that he has stated his principles "with a view to bringing into existence the maximum possible benefits consistent with the recognition that all are equally deserving of respect and fair consideration."[57] This comment once again discloses the dual concerns that have perennially emerged in discussions of triage: "maximum possible benefits" or utility and equal respect for persons in need or equality. Young calls his positon "egalitarian." But an analysis of his proposed principles shows that all five are basically concerned with utility in one form or another. Preserving, so far as possible, an equality of opportunity for all who are in need is not the first purpose of this position.

But equality of access to the scarce resources is the dominant concern of other ethicists who have written about the morality of triage. Once again, other principles may be incorporated, however implicitly, and various exceptions may be recognized. But the burden of proof is placed on anyone advocating a deviation from equality of opportunity. Ramsey's work is typical of this perspective. He advocates random selection (which he equates with queuing). But he assumes that the selections are made from "medically eligible" candidates.[58] Even so, he worries that estimates of medical suitability will incorporate hidden evaluations of general social value. And he reminds us that treatment of medically unpromising patients has sometimes been surprisingly successful. Nevertheless, he does not foreclose the possibility that the physician "who is forced to choose who lives, and who dies, does not act wrongly in proceeding on the optimum statistics."[59] What is more, Ramsey is willing to grant that in some exceptional circumstances when "a community have (or have been reduced to) a single focus or purpose and goal" candidates may be selected because of the socially valued function they can perform. Under such conditions, Ramsey grants the moral appropriateness of what we have called the principle of immediate usefulness. Thus, to take one of his examples, it would be justifiable to favor a physician in disaster triage because of the demands of the common good. Ramsey provides little help in defining what kinds of single purpose or goals would justifiably lead to evaluations of immediate social value. (Presumably he would rule out such goals as the establishment of a master race.) But it is clear that he sees such occasions as being rare exceptions, and his basic concern remains the preservation of fair equality of opportunity.

Dividing the triage proposals into two camps, utilitarian and egalitarian, is in some ways too neat and too simple. Some modes of allocation do not fit agreeably in either category (although, of course, it is nearly always possible to provide a utilitarian rationale for most any principle). Distributing scarce resources as a just reward for past meritorious actions is one such approach which does not fit neatly. Making resources available only to those who can pay is another. But no ethicist has been known to make either money or merit the *central* concern for triage. And several have rejected both notions. Thus, even though utility and equality may fail to cover all triage principles, they nevertheless represent the two most fundamental perspectives, which characterize the various proposals offered to date.

Childress suggests that such basic differences in perspective may be due to the differences in situations which the ethicists take to be paradigmatic. In his words:

> These different systems of allocation often rest on different models of the cases that the system will handle. Should the system be designed for the 'hard' or the 'easy' cases? And which side should bear the burden of proof? How heavy should the burden be for those who would argue for exceptions?[60]

Childress goes on to suggest that one who stresses the importance of social worth evaluations may simply be thinking of a different kind of "typical" case than one who favors strict equality.

Some evidence for the truth of Childress' analysis comes from the foregoing discussion of principles in the light of our two prismatic cases. It was unusual to find that a principle would be more appropriate in one case than another. For example, the principle of immediate usefulness is far more likely to seem plausible for disaster triage than for the allocation of artificial hearts. But having said this, we have hardly resolved the fundamental differences between utilitarian and egalitarian approaches to triage. The differences in these perspectives cannot all be attributed to the different kinds of cases taken as models. Even if the same cases were understood as typical, some ethicists would almost certainly favor a basically utilitarian position while others would reject just such a position and advocate some more strictly egalitarian approach.

We return, then, to our earlier question: Is any ranking of the principles more just than another? There are obvious perplexities and obstacles to assigning such an order to any set of moral principles. But even if it is not within reach to give a complete ranking in ordinal fashion, it may still be possible to rule out some approaches as unjust. For assistance in this endeavor we turn to the work of John Rawls. No other major work on justice in recent times has gone so far in attempting to order principles of justice for social institutions.

VI Justice as Fairness

IN THE PRECEDING CHAPTERS, two fundamentally different approaches to triage have been discussed, one stressing utility and the other equality. In general, the utilitarian emphasis has held sway both in thought and in practice. But important egalitarian challenges have been mounted, especially with regard to the distribution of scarce new technologies.

These two distinct approaches will hardly seem unfamiliar to moral philosophers concerned with justice. The relationship of utility to equality has continued to be an important issue in many discussions of distributive justice. It is not uncommon for such discussions to analyze the meaning of utility and equality and then prescribe some balance between the two.[1] The ideal is often portrayed as a social system that would achieve maximum increases in average utility while reducing to a minimum any inequalities in human rights or levels of well-being. Thus, both utility and equality are taken to be "first principles" (a designation that may be shared with a number of other principles as well).

Since it is generally recognized that such principles may be in conflict, the maintenance of equilibrium becomes a major theoretical problem. For example, it is often argued that there must be trade-offs between utility and equality; increments in one are to be balanced against reductions in the other, generally in some intuitive manner.[2] The formulas for balancing may be rather elaborate. But, characteristically, final decisions are left to an intuitive weighing of first principles. Such balancing of equality and utility, as we have seen, has also been reflected in triage proposals.

But the treatise on justice that unquestionably has provoked the most sustained and vigorous discussion in recent years purports to go beyond an intuitive balancing of utility and equality. In *A Theory of Justice*, John Rawls argues that a resuscitated and refurbished contract theory can better represent our considered judgments about social justice. Although Rawls does not claim that all intuitive balancing can be eliminated from any moral theory,[3] he argues that contract theory can help to minimize reliance on intuition by providing a more systematic way to check the coherence of our moral convictions.

As would be expected, Rawls's theory has met with a wide range of responses. It has befuddled, annoyed, convinced, exhausted, and in some cases simply bored its readers. But few have called the theory unimportant.[4] Indeed, seldom has a philosophical work's significance been so readily certified by its most strident critics. As one of those critics comments, Rawls has produced "a work that anyone in [the] future who proposed to deal with any of the topics it touches must first come to terms with if he expects the scholarly community to take him seriously."[5]

I believe that Rawls's effort is not only important but also may serve to enlighten us about justice in triage. But the decision to examine triage in the light of Rawls's work is not made without a keen sense of the numerous difficulties in such an undertaking. There are those, for example, who argue that the idea of contract is inappropriate for the delivery of health care.[6] And, it must be granted, few discussions of the delivery of health care have been structured in terms of Rawls's theory.[7] Even if one agrees that some version of contract theory may serve as a basis for an understanding of just health care delivery, the practice of triage raises special problems. Some of these will be addressed in the course of the following discussion. But, in spite of the obstacles, it will be argued that Rawls's theory, when suitably qualified and extended, enables us better to assess the justness of specific triage proposals.

One of Rawls's critics has suggested that future philosophers of justice "must either work within Rawls' theory or explain why not."[8] There is, however, another alternative. One may use Rawls's work to illuminate the problem under discussion and in turn allow the problem to suggest additions, modifications, or extensions of the theory. It is in this manner that this chapter proceeds with a discussion of triage "within" the framework of Rawls's theory of justice as fairness.

Because Rawls's views have been so often and so widely discussed by other scholars, a comprehensive summary should be unnecessary. The purpose here is to focus on the main features of Rawls's position, especially those most important for the discussion of triage. Criticisms of the theory will emerge later. It is hoped that this process will then enable us to select, reject, and order the various approaches to triage from the perspective of Rawls's theory of justice as fairness.

Rawls's Theory of Justice

In order to derive principles of social justice, Rawls presents his well-known heuristic strategem called the "original position."[9] Rawls asks his readers to imagine a scene in which a group of people have been gathered for the purpose of establishing a system of procedural justice that is as "fair" as possible. The decision makers are rational, in the sense that they can fit means to ends, and they are self-interested. They are also free and equal. In all these features, the original position resembles the fictional assemblies of the classical social contract theories. But Rawls introduces a novel restriction.

The contractors do not know how any of the proposed alternatives will affect their own particular interests. In order to insure impartiality, the participants are placed behind a "veil of ignorance"[10] and so cannot know any information about themselves as unique individuals. Nor do they have any class biases or particular philosophical perspectives. They do, of course, need to have a general understanding of the workings of human societies including, for example, some knowledge of political science, economics, and psychology. The contractors also need a knowledge of those social goods that all rational people can be expected to want. Among these "primary goods" Rawls includes rights and liberties, opportunities and powers, income and wealth, and the bases of self-respect.[11] But specific information about the deliberators' own traits, such as intelligence, economic status, and individual life plans, are excluded.

The impartiality this conception of the original position is intended to guarantee is certainly not unique to Rawls. Moral philosophers have often invented Universal Lawgivers, Ideal Observers, or Sympathetic Spectators to serve as imaginary aids in deriving universalizable and impartial principles.[12] But Rawls believes that the original position with its veil of ignorance succeeds in important areas where these other models fail. Most significantly, the impartial spectator theories do not take seriously enough the distinctions between people. Such theories lend themselves to the support of certain aspects of utilitarianism which, Rawls charges, cannot be reconciled with our considered moral judgments. The vision of the impartial spectator is prone to reduce moral decisions to questions of efficient operation of the social system. By conflating the desires of all persons in the society and by adopting the singular goal of maximizing aggregate utility, individual rights and the principles of justice, which should have overriding importance, are demoted to the level of numerous other factors that are weighed in the calculations of the greatest net balance of satisfaction. The original position, on the other hand, retains the morally significant distinctions between individuals while insuring the impartiality of the resultant principles.

As an expository device, Rawls' hypothetical original position also serves another important goal: simplifying the choice of principles of social justice. This is accomplished by posing the problem of selection in terms of rational prudence. Thus, the complexities of social choice are exchanged for the more reliable judgments of self-interest by a rational agent. Once again, the intuitive idea is certainly not entirely novel. After all, Jesus' Golden Rule admonishes persons to consult their own interests in order to generalize principles of treatment for others.[13] But the original position is intended to eliminate the problems of idiosyncratic choices by limiting the knowledge of the decision makers. Moreover, this conception has the advantage of making weaker assumptions about the participants. In particular, they may be thought of as mutually disinterested rather than benevolent.[14] Because of the fair procedural restraints on the selection process, especially the veil of ignorance, rational prudence is sufficient to produce just principles.

In order to make Rawls's original position with its veil of ignorance seem somewhat less ethereal, perhaps an illustration taken from common childhood experience would prove useful. Most children are at times confronted with situations that call for the sharing of a desired object—a candy bar, for instance. Since "taking turns" with a candy bar is likely to be not only unfair but also impracticable, some other method of distribution must be found. The "tried and proven" method (which most of us remember from our own early encounters with fairness) is to let one child cut the candy and the other child distribute the two pieces. Ordinarily the procedure is considered fair and the outcome is mutually satisfactory.

The illustration is far from perfect. But many of the features of the original position can be seen. It must be assumed, for example, that both children like candy, are rational, and have the normal degree of self-interest. The one cutting the candy is behind the veil of ignorance to the extent that s/he does not know for certain which piece will be hers/his. The illustration is happily uncluttered by considerations such as whether the candy was intended as a reward for a task on which one child worked more diligently than the other. (More about merit later.) But under the stated conditions, what sort of division of the candy is it reasonable to expect? Obviously, the rational choice of a child who likes candy is to cut the bar in the middle. Given the nature of the case, an equal division of the goods is certain to become the first operating principle.

This illustration reveals some of the characteristics of decision making under conditions of uncertainty. In the now familiar language of game theory,[15] the children are involved in a zero-sum game. That is, what one child gains the other loses. The situation is strictly competitive. The sum of gains and losses equals zero. But suppose that the circumstances are changed to a non-zero-sum game. Let us say, for example, that the size of the candy bar may become larger if the children are willing to accept unequal shares. Imagine, as well, that an adult is doing the dividing, and as part of the bargain both children will get bigger shares than they would have with the smaller candy bar, but one of the children will get the larger of the two expanded shares. Both of the children understand the scheme for the division of the larger bar, but neither child knows which share will be his/hers when the distribution is made. The differences in the distributional schemes of the zero-sum and non-zero-sum situations can be represented in the following way:

Scheme I (zero-sum)	
Share for A	Share for B

Scheme II (non-zero-sum)	
Share for A	Share for B

Not knowing the outcome ahead of time, would it be rational for both children to agree to Scheme II? If one assumes the absence of envy and the presence of normal self-interest, the answer would appear to be yes.

The candy bar illustration gives a preview of the principles to which Rawls believes rational contractors would unanimously agree in the original position. Rawls claims that the participants would all support at least two fundamental principles:

> . . . The first requires equality in the assignment of basic rights and duties, while the second holds that social and economic inequalities, for example inequalities of wealth and authority, are just only if they result in compensating benefits for everyone and in particular for the least advantaged members of society.[16]

Thus, the two principles Rawls derives from the original position may be roughly designated as the "equality principle" (our term, not Rawls's) and the "difference principle." There is a basic presumption in favor of equality. (This result is hardly surprising, given the nature of the original position and the fact that the participants are portrayed as essentially similar to one another and protective of the interests considered to be most important to all human beings.) If there are to be exceptions to equal treatment, they must bear the burden of proof in a special way: within a reasonable time frame, inequalities must literally work out for the good of everyone, especially the least advantaged.

These principles are restated in many forms, and many refined nuances are added throughout Rawls's work. Eventually, the principle of strict equality refers to political liberties and the rights of equal citizenship. The second principle is split to include a principle of equal opportunity and the difference principle. A simplified version of what amounts to three distinct principles can be stated in their ranked order as follows:[17]

I. Each person has an equal right to the most extensive liberties compatible with similar liberties for all.

IIa. Social and economic inequalities are attached to offices and positions open to all under fair equality of opportunity.

IIb. Social and economic inequalities are arranged so that they achieve the greatest benefit for the least advantaged.

This version of the principles is intended to apply to a specially restricted vision of society. Stated in this manner, Rawls argues that the principles are constitutive of a "perfectly just order" under "ideal" conditions.[18] Each person in such a society, it is assumed, will act in accordance with the principles and support just social institutions. Thus, the principles as given in the above order are for what Rawls chooses to call "strict compliance" theory. Although the members of society are assumed to have conflicts of interest, they are also expected to have a basic identity of interests stemming from their understanding that cooperative endeavor will be advantageous for all members. This cooperation takes place in circumstances of moderate scarcity.[19] Thus, there is the need to cooperate and the resources are not so scarce as to threaten the value of the cooperative efforts. And the participants have a sense of justice that predisposes them to respect the principles of justice.

Under such "ideal" conditions, Rawls believes the principles would be ranked in the order given above. Rational deliberators would give the principle of equal liberty top priority. This principle would have to be satisfied before any others became obligatory. The contractors would be unwilling, for example, to trade their liberty for greater average utility. This is so, Rawls argues, becauses liberty is necessary for the full enjoyment of other goods, regardless of one's life plan.[20] And some other goods, especially the good of self-respect, are best guaranteed by granting equal liberty to all citizens of the society. Rawls recognizes that there may be societies in which the level of economic development is so low that the citizens would be preoccupied with the necessities for survival and the priority of equal liberty would not yet have emerged. But it is argued that once the basic needs of a society's members can be met, equal liberty would become the "chief regulative interest" of the rational contractors.[21]

Second place in Rawls's serial ranking goes to fair equality of opportunity.[22] This principle takes priority over any strategies for maximizing utility and it also comes before the difference principle. Rawls grants that having favored positions open to all might lead to less than maximum average utility and/or less than a maximum minimum. But he contends that rational deliberators would not accept restrictions on fair equality of opportunity for these reasons. Rather, the participants would insist on the priority of equality of opportunity not only because they would want the chance to enjoy the external rewards of the favored positions (for example, wealth and privilege but also because they would desire the opportunities for self-realization that such positions would afford.[23]

The concept of fair equality of opportunity is obviously subject to numerous interpretations.[24] For example, having preferred offices open to *everyone* might mean that the positions are granted to the winners of a lottery, or on the basis of some rotational scheme, or through fair competition. But, as Rawls explains the principle, "open to all" means equal opportunities for those who have similar talents and motivations. In his words:

> [A]ssuming that there is a distribution of natural assets, those who are at the same level of talent and ability, and have the same willingness to use them, should have the same prospects of success regardless of their initial place in the social system, that is, irrespective of the income class into which they are born. In all sectors of society there should be roughly equal prospects of culture and achievement for everyone similarly motivated and endowed.[25]

Thus, in justice as fairness, equality of opportunity is understood in essentially competitive terms. This position is obviously not free of problems when viewed in the light of Rawls's larger theory. One of the main tenets of justice as fairness is that we should seek a conception of justice that "nullifies the accidents of natural endowment and the contingencies of social circumstance as counters in quest for political and economic advantage. . . ."[26] And yet Rawls readily admits that familial and cultural impingements may decisively affect a person's motivation or talents and thus his/her ability to compete for the favored positions. Nevertheless, Rawls argues that equality of opportunity does not necessitate attempts to overcome all of the potentially disadvantaging effects of a person's past. What the principle prohibits is the arbitary exclusion of any person from society's preferred positions which s/he has the motivation to seek and the ability to fill.

There are, then, practical limitations to fair equality of opportunity, and these may seem troublesome to a liberal, egalitarian theory. But Rawls believes that viewing the principle of equal opportunity in competitive terms should not be particularly problematic in justice as fairness. This is because the principle of equal opportunity is coupled with the difference principle, which works to the benefit of the least advantaged and thus tends to equalize opportunities in the long run. Thus, the difference principle has some of the same effects as a principle of redress.[27] And the people in the least advantaged position (who, in any event, are assumed not to be envious) will tend to be satisfied with the potential for benefits arising from application of the difference principle. They will not be prone to complain about the social or personal obstacles that may have hindered their ability to compete for the favored positions.

After equal liberty and fair equality of opportunity have been established, the difference principle comes into force. According to this principle, inequalities must work to the advantage of the least advantaged in the long run. Why should the participants in the original position unanimously agree to maximize the minimum payoff (or, in Rawls's terms, choose the "maximin rule") instead of accepting some other strategy such as maximizing average utility? Rawls does not argue that rational decision-making under conditions of uncertainty would always lead to this choice.[28] But he contends that the special restrictions placed on the original position and its contractors would lead to choosing the maximin rule. The same conditions that permit the original position with its veil of ignorance to aid in the selection of just principles also give the deliberators an aversion to risk and a wariness about probability calculations. This is because they realize that they may be one of those in the least advantaged positions when the veil or ignorance is lifted. Moreover, it must be remembered, they are not envious and care little about the primary goods they may receive above the maximum possible minimum.[29] The contractors are unwilling to structure society (as Rawls says some utilitarians might) so that prosperity may be purchased for the majority at the expense of having a few serfs or slaves. Indeed, it is precisely this kind of result that the maximin rule is designed to prevent.

The principles in their serial ranking, as just described, are intended to represent the chief features of social justice for *ideal* conditions. But Rawls grants, of course, that life in any actual society is likely to be far from the conditions presented in his ideal theory. Not everyone will comply with the principles. And factors such as the "accidents of nature" may add to the difficulties and complexities of social cooperation along the lines of Rawls's theory. For these less favorable conditions, Rawls says it may be necessary to relinquish the order of the principles just outlined in favor of a more general conception derived from the original position. He states this general conception in the following words:

> All social primary goods—liberty and opportunity, income and wealth, and the bases of self-respect—are to be distributed equally unless an unequal distribution of any or all of these goods is to the advantage of the least favored.[30]

Rawls knows that it will often be the case that no perfectly just solutions are available. "In practice we must usually choose between several unjust, or second best, arrangements; and then we look to nonideal theory to find the least unjust scheme."[31] When the best we can do is less than a completely just solution, we still may receive guidance from the general conception. And even in such nonideal circumstances, we should be reluctant to wholly discard the priority rules for the specific principles because they may assist us in deciding which problems to work on first.

Rawls's work is long and elaborate. It is hoped, however, that the fundamental sense of the theory has been conveyed in a way that will permit us to pursue the discussion of triage in the light of his system. But first there are some important obstacles to this task which must be addressed.

Problems of Fit

Of the difficulties that complicate fitting the discussion of triage within a Rawlsian framework, the following are sufficiently important to require comment before attempting to extract the implications of Rawls's work for triage decision making.

1. *Justice as fairness is conceived for conditions of moderate scarcity and not the dire scarcity of triage.* Following Hume, Rawls describes the context of justice in terms of moderate scarcity.[32] A superabundance of every desired good, Rawls agrees, would make principles of justice otiose. And if scarcities are so severe that social cooperation would be rendered unfruitful, then principles of justice also would become inapplicable. Moderate scarcity, however, makes social cooperation both possible and attractive. Goods are plentiful enough so that schemes of social cooperation are advantageous. But since it is impossible to satisfy all human interests, principles must be developed to handle competing claims.

At this point, only a few comments need to be added to our earlier discussion of Hume. The main point is this. The dire scarcities of triage situations are relatively isolated in time, or place, or scope, or perhaps all three. This means that triage conditions generally would not be expected to jeopardize the cooperative ventures of the society. An exception (of short duration) might be the natural disaster represented in the first of the two prismatic cases. But the question in such circumstances is not whether the principles of *justice* cease to be morally relevant but whether sufficient *order* can be maintained so that any scheme of allocation can be initiated.

The kind of scarcities which, according to Hume (and apparently Rawls), would vitiate the principles of justice are those which would affect the whole society and reduce its members to a competitive struggle for survival. The assumption is that moderate scarcity must prevail throughout most of the society most of the time in order for the principles of justice to be effective. Or as Rawls says, "moderate scarcity [is] understood to cover a *wide range* of situations."[33] Though he does not say so explicitly, it appears safe to infer that Rawls means that some goods may be overabundant and some may be tragically scarce so long as moderate scarcity is the predominant condition. This interpretation is further bolstered by the fact that justice as fairness is concerned with the basic structure of the whole society and not isolated situations (a problem that will be taken up momentarily).

Portraying the contractors as primarily concerned with conditions of moderate scarcity does not prevent their consideration of restricted occurrences of dire scarcity. There is nothing about the scarcities illustrated in the two prismatic cases that would preclude rational deliberations by participants in the original position. The fact that ordinary people have already conducted discussons about and planning for the allocation of scarce life-saving goods for both prismatic cases is evidence that such reflection is not only feasible but is also considered important. In any event, it is not the first aim of a theory of justice to determine how far it is likely that just principles will actually be applied.

2. *The principles of justice as fairness are intended for the basic structure of society and its major institutions and not primarily for microallocation decisions such as triage.* The question is: How applicable are general principles of social justice to the small-scale distributional problems of triage, which affect only a limited segment of the society?

Social justice, according to Rawls, is concerned with the way "major social institutions distribute fundamental rights and duties and determine the division of advantages from social cooperation."[34] As noted earlier, Rawls includes the political organization, the major economic arrangements, and the established social practices such as the monogamous family under the rubric of "major institutions." An institution is described as a "public system of rules which defines offices and positions with their rights and duties, powers and immunities, and the like."[35] These dominant practices affect the life prospects of every societal member in decisive ways.

Rawls does not include the medical care system in his list of major social institutions. (More on this lacuna in a moment.) But there is little question that the organization of health care delivery in modern societies has become a major social institution by virtually any definition. As Jonsen and Hellegers aptly put it:

> Medicine has, in recent years, evolved from a practice, a
> private technical interaction between two parties, through a
> profession, a socially coherent, publicly recognized group that
> defines the conditions under which those private transactions
> take place, to an institution.[36]

The time when most questions of health care distribution
had to do with the way a private practitioner apportioned
his/her time and effort is gone. Modern medicine has become
an increasingly prominent sector in the overall economy of the
industrialized nations. Institutional features such as rapidly
increasing costs, the problems attending third-party payments,
and the maldistribution of personnel and facilities have made
the health care system the source of considerable social concern. As a social institution, the health care business has a
significant impact on a variety of public decisions that affect
other social institutions. Without question, the way the institution of medical care is organized has important consequences for the life prospects of society's members. Failure to
take into account the institutional nature of contemporary
health care delivery, as the authors just quoted point out, is
bound to lead to inept ethical analysis.

But even if it is agreed that the medical care system is a
social institution of great importance, this does not mean that
principles for the larger system all would be applicable in micro
situations. Triage, as we have presented it in this study, is concerned first of all with microallocation decisions, and not with
the health care institution as a whole. It is just this kind of
microallocation problem for which, as Rawls is careful to point
out, the principles of justice as fariness are not primarily
designed. In fact, Rawls says that we cannot assume that principles governing the basic structure will always be appropriate
for specific allocative problems.[37] To borrow a line from Wolff,
Rawls contends that the principles of justice as fairness are to
"apply to the broad, basic organization or institutional arrangement of society, not to every baseball team, stamp club,
and mom-and-pop grocery store."[38] And, we might add, not to
every triage plan.

Rawls has been criticized for abstracting the principles of
justice from the kinds of specific cases where questions of
justice often arise. Nozick, for example, wonders how we

could ever assay the sense of Rawls's principles without the benefit of micro test cases.

> For many of us, an important part of the process of arriving at what Rawls calls 'reflective equilibrium' will consist of thought experiments in which we try out principles in hypothetical microsituations. If, in our considered judgment, they don't apply there then they are not universally applicable.[39]

Nozick goes on to argue that it is difficult for us accurately to perceive a complex whole. Thus, we should not seek to derive most of our moral principles from attempts to view society as a whole. Rather, we should be willing to change our judgments about principles for the entire social structure by examining them in the light of principles "solidly founded at the micro level."[40]

In these contentions, Nozick is about half right.[41] It is literally true, of course, that a principle that does not work in some situations, no matter how isolated, is not "*universally* applicable." It is also true that we may alter our intuitive principles for the larger society by "trying them out" in micro situations. Certainly this would be so if we found an exceedingly high proportion of counterexamples. But this process of testing must go in both directions. That is, we may also modify our principles for specific and limited circumstances by considering their cumulative effect when generalized. Moreover, even with such two-way testing, there is no reason to believe that the principles for micro situations will always resemble those for the whole social structure. It is obvious that just principles for, say, giving academic grades may not be suitable when applied to major social institutions distributing primary goods.[42] And just principles for the allocation of a limited number of artificial hearts to a specified group of candidates may be inappropriate for decision making about health care resources at the macroallocation level of national policy.

Rawls, as we have seen, is primarily concerned with the basic structure of society and the way the larger social institutions distribute primary goods. Of these goods, he concentrates on political rights and economic well-being.[43] But his attention to these factors does not prevent Rawls from applying his principles to other specific social practices. Consider, for example, his comments on the relation of the difference principle to education:

> [T]he difference principle would allocate resources in educa-
> tion, say, so as to improve the long-term expectation of the
> least favored. If this end is attained by giving more atten-
> tion to the better endowed, it is permissible; otherwise not.
> And in making this decision, the value of education should
> not be assessed solely in terms of economic efficiency and
> social welfare. Equally if not more important is the role of
> education in enabling a person to enjoy the culture of his
> society and to take part in its affairs, and in this way to pro-
> vide for each individual a secure sense of his own worth.[44]

Rawls does not talk about health care in the same manner. But there is no obvious reason why "health care" could not be substituted *mutatis mutandis* for "education" in the passage just quoted. No doubt, as broad principles for the major institu-tions including the health care system are applied to the more specific distributive problems such as triage, adaptations will have to be made in order to fit the circumstances. But, if Rawls is right, our judgments in these more limited situations often should be enlightened by the general conception of justice derived from the original position. Moreover, it should be noted, Rawls also claims that the process of selecting prin-ciples as described in justice as fairness should aid in choosing other principles of moral guidance, or what Rawls names "rightness as fairness."[45] My proposal, then, is that we at-tempt to discover what sort of guidance Rawls's contract theory has for the problems of triage, when the theory is ex-tended and adjusted to fit the nonideal, microallocation circumstances.

3. *In Rawls's theory, neither health nor health care are in-cluded among the social primary goods.* As seen earlier, Rawls concentrates his analysis primarily on wealth and liberty. He pays far less attention to other goods such as education. And he says almost nothing about health or health care.

One of the possible reasons for Rawls's near silence on the topic is that he considers health (along with vigor, in-telligence, and imagination) to be one of the *natural* primary goods. The acquisition of such natural goods, he says, is far less dependent on the basic structure of society than is the possession of the *social* primary goods such as liberty, wealth, and power.

To suggest that health is largely independent of the social structure is surely to ignore the complex interaction between health status and certain decidedly social factors such as levels of education and socioeconomic class.[46] But even if we permit Rawls to separate health in this way, it makes no sense to say that health *care* is independent of the basic social structure. In America today, for example, access to health care is affected by a multitude of social arrangements such as the fee-for-service delivery system. And, as argued above, the health care industry ranks among the most important of social institutions.

Of course, health care is not health, and there are those who would contend that the two are only slightly related.[47] It must be admitted, of course, that it is very difficult to define health in an objective way. But with virtually any definition of health, the current evidence seems to suggest that the relationship between health and medical care is far more tenuous than many would have thought. And it is surely an overstatement to say, as Green does in his discussion of Rawls and medical care, that "Modern medical technology, with its enormous preventative and therapeutic powers, renders almost archaic the notion that health depends on natural contingencies."[48]

Much of what we call health still depends largely on genetic endowment, personal habits, and the quality of the environment. But even if medicine has been erroneously portrayed as the guarantor of all health, it would be idle to suggest that health care should be considered an unimportant good by most people in society. This is particularly obvious for those medical treatments that are unquestionably life-saving. The chances of needing such care may be fairly remote; indeed, the vast majority of the populace may live their normal lives and need very little medical care. But, in many respects, human beings are all behind the veil of ignorance when it comes to the need for health care. A life-threatening disease may be statistically rare; but the disease may tend to afflict people in a random way. People generally do not know which maladies, if any, they will have. Thus, even if health care can only occasionally retrieve health or postpone death, such care is a good that rational people would not treat lightly, especially rational people with a strong aversion to risk. And such health *care* is a primary *social* good made available in modern societies by a highly complex social institution. Green is right: "Despite Rawls, then, health care ought to be considered a primary social good in his terms, and ought to be directly considered by a theory of justice."[49]

Regardless of Rawls's reasons for omitting health care from his list of primary social goods, rational contractors should consider health care to be among those goods a person wants "whatever else s/he wants." And life-saving health care would have to rank close to liberty as one of those primary goods that generally takes priority because, if needed, such care must be obtained before most other goods can be enjoyed.[50]

It must be said, however, that this strategy of relating health care to Rawls's theory by incorporating health care in Rawls's list of primary social goods is not without problems and has been challenged by Daniels.[51] It is not enough, according to Daniels, to argue that health care is an especially important good. So are food and shelter. But, Daniels argues, the inclusion of such goods in the catalogue of *primary* social goods would defeat Rawls's purpose. The list is supposed to be so general that it covers the goods wanted by all members of society regardless of their special circumstances. And the exchange value of income and wealth is supposed to take care of the particular needs unique to any individual. Thus, in Daniels's view, the inclusion of health care would be a significant change in Rawls's theory of social primary goods.

But Daniels himself recognizes that health care may differ from most other basic goods in important ways. As a rule, the exchange value of wealth will take care of a person's needs for such things as food and shelter. These needs are relatively equal and constant among society's members. But this is hardly the case with health care, especially life-saving health care. Needs for such care generally arise unpredictably and, given modern medical technology, can be prohibitively expensive for the individual. Any theory of justice that fails to take into account such special dimensions of health care is likely to be found inadequate. And from the perspective of rational contractors, any list of primary social goods would be incomplete without the inclusion of at least life-saving health care.[52]

4. *It is difficult to determine the constituency for whom the principles of contract theory have force.* This is a problem for any theory of justice. Formulating solutions that are free of arbitrariness is not easily done and, in the history of the concept of justice, the results are not particularly reassuring. Great moral philosophers, it seems, frequently developed worthy principles of justice only to exclude classes of people from the principles' jurisdiction in ways that now appear downright unjust.[53]

In modern health care, the problems of constituency are largely the by-products of the institutionalization of scientific medicine. When a lone practitioner pursued his or her art within an easily identifiable, cohesive community, few questions of constituency arose. But today the complex interaction of institutions which finance and control the research, development, and eventual utilization of medical technology make the concept of constituency difficult to analyze.

Put simply, the question is: Who should be included in the basic reference group for which the rights and duties of social justice are considered binding? In the case of triage, this basic question should be distinguished from the more specific questions about criteria for patient selection. Obviously, the difference is more one of degree than of kind. To answer the constituency question is, in a sense, already to take the first step toward a triage decision. But before one can consider the moral relevance of selection criteria such as parental role, medical success, or general social worth, it is necessary to set the outermost boundaries of the population to be considered. For the sake of analysis, we can divide the problem into two parts: the limits of being, and the limits of society.

The Limits of Being

Traditionally, the constituency of justice has been limited to humans.[54] Of late, however, increased attention has been given to the putative rights of animals,[55] and many of the moral distinctions between animals and humans have been challenged. Even Nozick, for example, says: "Once they exist,

127

animals too may have claims to certain treatment."⁵⁶ The question, then, is: What attribute, if any, justifies granting the protection of the princples of justice to all human progeny but not to the nonhuman creatures of the world?

For Rawls, the key attribute is the capacity for moral personality. By this he means the ability to develop a sense of justice and have a conception of one's own good.⁵⁷ Rawls offers an aphorism for this conception of constituency: "Those who can give justice are owed justice."⁵⁸ The grounds for this maxim lie at the heart of the contract theory. Free and equal persons, each deserving of the others' respect, join together in cooperative endeavors, producing goods, which should then be distributed through social institutions in accordance with just principles. Participants must be rational and capable of a sense of justice so that they can share in the bargaining and support the just institutions that result.

Rawls protects this view of constituency against a number of obvious criticisms. For example, he includes children by arguing that the capacity for moral personality should be regarded as a *potential* for an understanding of one's own good and a sense of justice.⁵⁹ He also guards against the criticism that basing justice on the capacity for moral personality would imply stronger claims to justice for those with a keener sense of justice. Rawls contends that moral personality is a "range property."⁶⁰ The capacity may be greater or smaller, but once a certain minimum is met, equal rights to justice are established.

But what about those who are, so far as can be determined, permanently incapable of moral personality even at some minimal level? Rawls excludes animals,⁶¹ but he is unwilling to exclude those human beings who, through accident or defect, appear not to have the capacity for self-awareness or a sense of justice. His argument on this point is, however, somewhat inconclusive. Moral capacity is sufficient grounds for equal justice. But is this attribute also *necessary*? One would be prone to think, given the rest of Rawls's theory, that the answer would be yes. But Rawls leaves the queston aside. It is better, he argues, to assume that the minimal conditions are always satisfied by all human beings.⁶² Since the vast majority do have the capacity for moral personality, those few who may be exceptions do not represent a serious practical problem. In any case, he asserts, it would be imprudent to withhold justice from the exceptional ones: "The risk to just institutions would be too great."[63]

The net effect of Rawls's argument is to include equally all human members of society within the constituency of justice. The majority are included because they are capable of giving justice, a minority because not to do so would unwisely jeopardize just institutions. Some may consider this to be an inadequate account of human equality. But, for the present, it can be said that this part of Rawls's theory does not pose any practical problems for triage decision making. The medical resources we have been discussing are representative of the products of social cooperation by human beings. Whether plasma, ambulance services, surgical techniques, or artificial hearts, such resources are made available by human beings for the purpose of alleviating human maladies. Such maladies afflict human beings rather indiscriminately. And it is reasonably safe to assume that the vast majority of those in need have what Rawls would call the minimum capacity for moral personality. Moreover, since Rawls does not leave us with the task of deciding which of the human progeny fall below this minimum, we may simply assume that all human beings in need within the society should be considered part of the basic constituency covered by the principles of justice.

The Limits of Society

Having settled on humans as the kind of beings to whom justice is owed, what are the boundaries of society within which just institutions are possible?

Among triage problems natural disasters have their own boundaries, and there are fewer questions about where to stop looking for candidates for the scarce resources.[64] But the problems of setting societal limits are more obvious and complicated for the artificial heart since it is likely to be needed by people throughout the world. At present, research and development are being conducted not only at a number of centers in the United States but also in several other nations.[65] There is sharing of information and, in some cases, hardware. The

United States, for example, has been engaged in a joint research program with the Soviet Union since 1974. Thus, if and when one nation succeeds in developing a clinically acceptable artificial heart, it will be at least partially the result of international efforts.

Another illustration of the problem and one response to it was provided by the selection committee for renal dialysis at Seattle's Swedish Hospital. The committee, it will be remembered, decided not to consider any candidates from outside the state of Washington.[66] The rationale was that Washington State taxpayers had helped to finance the development of the dialysis technology. Thus, it was felt, Washington citizens should be considered the center's constituency and have first claim on the services. Of course, money to support the Washington research had also come from other sources, including the federal government.[67] And an uneasiness with the decision to limit the candidates to Washington residents was expressed by one committee member: "This was arbitrary . . . but we had to start somewhere!"[68] It might be said that the committee had already started "somewhere" when they limited their deliberation to human beings, to citizens of the United States, and so forth. But the committee's decision reveals the need to confine the distributive problem to some identifiable and, presumably, justifiable group. The decision also illustrates some of the factors Rawls includes in his account of the circumstances of social justice.

For Rawls, the place to begin is with a society of free and equal citizens who have the capacity for moral personality and occupy a definite geographical location.[69] Participants must constitute a society in some distinct geographical area so that cooperative efforts are possible. But more important than geography is the establishment of common social institutions such as a political constitution. Given the present realities in the world, the primary concept of constituency that emerges from Rawls's account is that of a nation-state within which all human beings have equal citizenship and thus are governed and protected by the principles of justice. Rawls says very little about international relations, but when he does suggest using the original position to generate principles of international justice, the contractors are portrayed as representatives of their various nations, not as citizens of the world.[70] His discussion of matters such as majority rule, civil disobedience, and the political constitution all imply that "society" in his theory, at least in today's world, means the nation-state.

In the ensuing discussion of triage from the perspective of contract theory, Rawls's view of the societal limits of constituency is adopted. The constituents are assumed to be members of a society with common social institutions, including a political constitution. This means that no attempt is made to address the problems of international justice. At its largest, the constituency is assumed to be a society of human beings within the boundaries of a sovereign state. Of course, most triage decisions, at least as the expression is used here, are not national, let alone international, in scope. Rather, they are limited primarily to local communities and local institutions. Although it is not inconceivable that national guidelines would be established for the allocation of a scarce medical resource, the actual decisions probably would have to be made at the local level. In any event, setting the societal limits in terms of the citizenry of the nation-state is a way of establishing the farthest boundaries of constituency for purposes of the present discussion.

In some respects, this choice of constituency is more pragmatic than principled. And the choice is made with the awareness of certain incongruities. For example, Rawls insists that principles of justice must be both general and universal.[71] In order to satisfy the formal criterion of generality, principles must not refer to particular individuals or groups. To be universal, principles must be capable of having everyone comply without being self-defeating, contradictory, or inconsistent. Now it may be possible behind the veil of ignorance to state a principle such as fair equality of opportunity so that it applies to any (as yet unnamed) society. But is generality still possible once the veil is lifted? Are favored positions in, say, Canada then supposed to be open to all Canadians or rather to all human beings?

One possible, contract-theory justification for having the positions open only to Canadians might be that such positions

131

are part of Canadian social institutions, which have resulted from Canadian cooperation. But, given an increasingly interdependent world, how convincing is this argument when applied to the problems of access to scarce medical resources? As mentioned earlier, development of medical technology, such as the artificial heart, is more and more the result of international cooperation. Thus, providing equal access to scarce artificial hearts for all those who can claim to have supported social institutions that have either directly or indirectly contributed to the development of the devices almost would certainly require some international policy.

The trouble is that there appears to be little or no practical way, at present, to implement principles of social justice at the international level. For example, there is no doubt that the demand for some sophisticated and scarce medical resources frequently transcends national boundaries.[72] But international institutions necessary for a just distribution of such resources are, for the most part, lacking. Even within the nation-state, there are likely to be problems with regional and institutional boundaries.[73] There are also likely to be problems with maldistribution of the resources available within the nation.[74] But, presumably, most sovereign states have some social mechanisms for addressing such problems and for attempting solutions. It is primarily for this reason that the discussion focuses on institutions within the nation-state.

Other problems between Rawls's theory and the circumstances of triage will emerge later. But the task now at hand is the consideration of triage from the perspective of the rational contractors as qualified by the forgoing provisions.

VII   Triage and Justice

THE TIME HAS COME to assess the various approaches to triage in the light of Rawls's theory of justice as fairness as qualified in the previous discussion. Life-saving health care is considered one of the primary social goods, and the health care system is viewed as a major social institution. The rational contractors are imagined to be selecting just principles for the allocation of life-saving resources in relatively isolated situations of dire scarcity.

The Equality Principle and Triage for the Artificial Heart

As noted earlier, the general conception that, according to Rawls, would be accepted by rational contractors has a basic presumption in favor of equality. The participants would subscribe to an equal distribution of social primary goods unless inequality would be to the advantage of the least favored. Thus inequalities must bear a heavy burden of proof: it must be reasonable to expect that any inequalities would maximize the minimum benefits. If this could not be demonstrated, the negotiators would opt for equality. They would not settle for less, and they know that it would be pointless to demand more. They would be uninterested in calculating probabilities of maximum average utility because their first concern would be to protect against the worst possible outcomes. The reason for their conservative attitude is that they would know that the goods in question are of paramount importance to any life plan they might have. They would, therefore, find it intolerable to take losses at the low end of any distributive scheme. And they would be unwilling to vote for gains in efficiency unless the added efficiency somehow improved the position of the worst off.

Agreement on equality would be particularly obvious if the contractors were considering a zero-sum situation. By definition, it would be impossible under these conditions to increase the minimum benefits by giving more to the better off. What would be given to better-off person A simply would not be available for distribution to worse-off person B. And nothing A could do, short of transferring some of the goods to B, would improve B's lot. In this situation, rational contractors, at least conservative ones of the Rawlsian variety, would select a strictly equal distribution. If improved efficiency resulting in increased benefits for the worst off were impossible, the only way to be *certain* of the best minimum would be to insist on equality. Otherwise, one could not be sure, when the veil of ignorance is lifted, that his or her position would not be among the worst off.

Allocation of the artificial heart would represent many of the characteristics of a zero-sum situation. If only four artificial hearts were available, for instance, and if ten patients were known to need the units, the circumstances would be strictly competitive in that the gain of one would be the loss of some other. It would be, by hypothesis, impossible to manufacture and implant the needed number of new devices in time to save all ten potential recipients. Nor would the chances of survival for the six not selected be improved if the four recipients had some special skills, even the skills of highly trained medical personnel. Thus, no alternative distribution would be likely to increase the maximum possible number of lives saved, though, of course, some alternative distributions might better assure the effective use of the available devices so that the maximum number could actually be reached.

Under these circumstances, it would be rational to select a principle of equal *access* as the basic principle on which to conduct triage. Given the nature of the goods being distributed and the conditions of dire scarcity, an equal distribution obviously would be impossible in the most absolute sense. Assuming that the four available devices were put to use, four of the candidates would get all of the goods, six would get nothing. The rational choice for the contractors would be to guarantee equal access to the obtainable units because, barring overriding concerns for efficiency (which we will discuss momentarily), no other approach would improve the contractors' chances of being recipients if they were among those in need.

The contractors would interpret equal access, in this case, to mean equal chances of being a recipient for each person who needs and wants the scarce resources. It would be irrational, of course, to include in the group of candidates those who do not actually need the resources in order to continue life. The contractors would be unwilling to reduce their own prospects for life by including those who desire the resource for reasons less important than the saving of life. Unlike Rawls's competitive interpretation of equal opportunity for favored positions, the contractors would understand the principle, as applied to triage, first of all in terms of medical needs. That is, the basic "qualification" which would justify including a person in the group of candidates would be the need for the resources in order to prevent the harm of death.

In addition to needing the resources, equal access would be for those who choose to be considered candidates by expressing some desire for the scarce resources. The importance the contractors would give equal liberty would be sufficient to establish the right of a person *not* to be included among the candidates if she or he chooses not to be. But any indication that a person who needs the resources also wants them would be considered sufficient evidence of the person's choice to be included among the candidates.[1] Of course, it might be objected that according equal access to all the candidates in need would give the claims of the person who barely wants the resources the same weight as the claims of one who desperately wants the resources.[2] But the contractors would likely consider any expressed decision for seeking the resources to be adequate. There would be no accurate way to gauge the degree of desire for the resources. And, since it is reasonable to assume that most people wish to go on living, whatever else they might want, one person's expressed desire to seek the scarce life-saving resources should be considered *prima facie* equal to any other person's. Otherwise a person's candidacy for

135

the resources might depend on an ability to sound convincing—a possibility that the contractors would surely find unacceptable.

If the forgoing arguments are correct and the contractors would choose a basic principle of equal access, how would they evaluate the approaches to triage presented in the last two chapters? In a case such as the artificial heart, it might seem that most of the utilitarian princples would be quickly rejected. The contractors, it might be supposed, would then discuss which of the egalitarian approaches could best assure fair equality of access. But such an out-of-hand rejection of the utilitarian approaches would be too hasty. At the very least, it must be granted that some utilitarian approaches would be more attractive to the contractors than others.

Equal Access and Utilitarian Qualifications

The utilitarian principles that probably would be least appealing for selecting artificial heart recipients would be the principles of immediate usefulness (U-2), which would give priority to those with immediately needed skills; parental role (U-4), which would give priority to those functioning as parents; and general social value (U-5), which would give priority to those judged to have greater general worth to the society. For reasons given earlier, the principle of immediate usefulness probably would be judged inappropriate. Nothing about the recipients of artificial hearts (or, for that matter, most any conceivable new medical technology) would be of immediate use in saving the unchosen candidates.

The principle of general social value also would be unattractive. In the original position, the contractors would lack personal knowledge about their own competitive chances of success in any social-worth evaluation. Indeed, the provisions of the veil of ignorance are specifically designed to rule out such comparisons of social value. Justice as fairness is a conception that seeks to nullify the "accidents of natural endowment and the contingencies of social circumstance as counters in quest for political and economic [and, we might add, *medical*] advantage."[3] Giving priority to those judged to have greater general social value would not interest the participants because such an approach would not improve their chances of being recipients in any way that could be known to them. And even if favoring those of greater social worth could be shown to benefit the least advantaged in terms of some other good such as wealth, the participants would still be unimpressed. They would be unwilling to accept less than equal access to the scarce life-saving resources in trade for an increased minimum of other primary goods. Whatever the specific details of their life plans, they would know that the first condition would be life itself.

But would it not be rational to figure that one's own chances of needing the scarce resources probably would be very slim? A contractor then might be willing to favor using general social worth criteria on the grounds that society thus could be improved with only a very small chance of personal loss. In fact, just such an argument has been offered by Basson. He suggests that the argument would be convincing not only to a rational contractor but also to a person in the real world, even if she knew herself to be of little social worth:

> Even in the real world to which a claim about democracy would appeal, without any veil of ignorance, the rational person who ranks low on the social value scale should realize that while social value-oriented allocation diminished his access to scarce medical resources, this will be offset by the greater payoff to all members of society engendered by the practice of allocating medical resources to socially useful people.[4]

What Basson seems to ignore is that just this line or reasoning, with its implied calculations of probability, is supposed to be prevented in the original position. The contractors would not find it acceptable, for example, to allow even two percent of the population to be enslaved so that the vast majority could be better off. The fact that one's own chances of being a slave would be very small would not move the contractors to vote for the institution of slavery. Rawlsian contractors, with their attention fixed first of all on the prospects of the worst off, would reject this type of reasoning. Similarly, they would reject the argument that triage based on general social worth is desirable because of the potential for improving society and the low probability of being among those denied equal access to the resources.

The principle of parental role would likely cause the contractors more consternation. This is partly because of a provision Rawls sometimes adds to the original position. He says that the contractors *may* be viewed as parents. "[W]e may think of the parties as heads of families, and therefore as having a desire to further the welfare of their nearest descendants."[5] Although Rawls does not think it necessary to view the participants as family heads, he generally portrays them this way. And it is important at this point to consider Rawls's reasons for including this provision, because thinking of the contractors as heads of families obviously has implications for their deliberations about the principle of parental role.

It is clear that Rawls introduces the condition of family ties in order to solve the problems of justice between generations and *not* to give some special advantages to parents. Nevertheless, it must be said that having the participants think of themselves as heads of families could jeopardize the impartiality supposedly guaranteed by the veil of ignorance. In the case of triage, for example, would it not be perfectly rational for participants who know that they are heads of families to select principles favoring candidates with children?[6] After all, if the participants know general facts about society, they must know that some people are not heads of families. Since they know themselves to be heads of families, it would, therefore, be rational to exclude those without families and thus improve their own chances of being selected.

There are at least two ways out of this apparent dilemma. The first is to declare it a "non-problem." We might grant that giving the contractors the knowledge that they are heads of families would result in principles favoring parents (and their children). But we might say that such an outcome is precisely what we had in mind all along. Parents should be given priority as a matter of justice, and the original position has again proven its worth by producing another principle that squares with our considered judgments.

There are, however, some obvious problems with this approach. What is there about parenthood which makes it a morally relevant or, more precisely, a just-making consideration, especially when the stake is life? There are few, if any, characteristics that would clearly abrogate a human being's right to life. Being single or without children is certainly not among them. Thus it is not at all clear that adopting the principle of parental role is in harmony with our considered moral judgments.

If, as is more likely, it is argued that favoring parents is a way of maintaining the well-being of children and is thus a matter of justice for children, other complications arise. Not all parents are good ones. Some are child abusers; others abandon their children. So in order to know which parents are of sufficient quality to justify their receiving priority in triage, considerable information about the parents' characters and the quality of family relationships would have to be introduced. In the process, the veil of ignorance would become too thin and tattered to assure impartiality.

Another way out of the dilemma posed by the principle of parental role—a way, it would seem, more in harmony with the rest of Rawls's theory—would be to drop the conception of the contractors as heads of families. There is no question that being a parent creates certain special obligations. But, generally speaking, these are obligations between parents and children. They are not obligations of a supposedly impartial third party (or group of rational contractors). Viewing the contractors as heads of families may help Rawls solve the problem of justice between generations,[7] but the price for this solution is too high. The impartiality of the original position is seriously undermined.

It still may be argued, of course, that children should receive some special protection because of their vulnerability. It does seem plausible to say that rational prudence would prompt the contractors to select principles to provide for children's special needs. Such a decision would stem from a concern for the particular needs of children, and not from the more utilitarian concern of the greatest good for the greatest number of family members. With regard to triage, the contractors probably would want to make provision for the care of children whose parents might not be selected as recipients of the scarce resources. But this is not the equivalent of giving parents priority in triage. Rather, each contractor probably would say something like this: "To be a child whose parent dies for lack of medical care would certainly be tragic. And, if I were such a child, I would want some special provisions made for my care. But what if I discover that I am a single person in need of the scarce resources? The regrets of losing a parent would not be the same as the regrets of not being selected if I find that I am one of the triage candidates. Thus, on balance, it is more important to me to guarantee equality of access to the scarce resources."

There remain two utilitarian principles that deserve evaluation from the perspective of the original position: the principle of medical success (U-1), which calls for giving priority to those with the best chances for a good medical outcome, and the principle of conservation (U-3), which prescribes priority for those requiring proportionately smaller amounts of the resources. Both may be viewed as principles of efficiency designed to save the largest possible number of lives. To the extent that such principles are applicable, the circumstances bear less resemblance to a zero-sum situation. The way the resources are allocated may affect the number of lives saved. This obviously does not always mean an increase in the maximum number of lives that potentially may be saved. In the case of the artificial heart, for example, that absolute maximum is likely to be fixed by the number of available units. But in such cases an efficiency principle such as the principle of medical success may serve to decrease the actual number of deaths.

The principle of medical success, when interpreted to mean the probability of sustaining life, has not been rejected by anyone known to have discussed triage. But the question now is: would such a principle be acceptable to the contract participants? Any attempt to answer the question inevitably leads us further into such perplexing aspects of Rawls's theory as the contractors' attitudes toward probability calculations and risk aversion.

Rawls's contractors, it will be remembered, are wary of probability calculations.[8] For example, they are unwilling to accept the principle of insufficient reason. That is, when in doubt about the probabilities of various outcomes because of lack of information, the contractors refuse to follow one of the commonly accepted tenets of decision theory and "take their chances" by assigning equal probabilities to the different potentialities. Rather, the contractors constantly seek to assure the highest possible minimum. When stripped of almost innumerable side issues, the reason Rawls has the contractors assume this rather conservative attitude toward risk is to prevent them from selecting one of the maximizing strategies of utilitarianism rather than his principle of maximin.[9] And the fundamental reason for guarding against utilitarian princples is that Rawls believes that utilitarianism might permit morally intolerable losses of primary goods for a few people in order to maximize the good for others.

Suppose we grant that it is ordinarily necessary to include the features of risk aversion and a tendency to discount probability calculations in order to avoid unacceptable utilitarian consequences and guarantee the maximin strategy. Nevertheless, these provisions would not be necessary in the same way when selecting principles of efficiency for the extraordinary circumstances of triage. The worst outcome in triage is death due to not receiving some necessary but scarce resource. There is not way to "maximin" except to maximize the probability of saving the greatest possible number of lives. For the contractors (especially conservative, risk-averting Rawlsian contractors), to do otherwise would be irrational.

Since the worst outcome is avoidable death, most any strategy that would decrease the chances of this untoward eventuality would gain immediate acceptance by the deliberators. For example, if the contractors were considering principles for the distribution of some scarce new medical technology such as the artifitical heart, and if the principle of medical success were proposed, each contractor could reason something like this: "I know that there may not be enough life-saving resources to go around. I do not know if I will be among those needing the resources. But I do know that some of the potential recipients have very poor chances of medical success while others have very good chances. Giving priority to those with markedly better chances is likely to result in the lowest possible proportion of lives lost. Since I wish to guard against the worst outcome, which is death, and since I lack any further information about my own status, it is rational for me to vote for the principle of medical success."

It should be noted that the willingness to consider probabilities in this case does not interfere with impartiality. The veil of ignorance is still intact. What is more, risk calculations do not necessarily lead away from maximin selections. Indeed, some kinds of probability considerations obviously would be essential in order to arrive at maximin strategies.[10]

A line of reasoning similar to that just developed for the principle of medical success would also lead the contractors to accept the principle of conservation. Because of its indivisibility, the artificial heart is not the best case to illustrate the point. But other variables, such as the time of medical personnel, might be subject to conservation so that additional lives could be saved. Again the concern would be to keep the probable proportion of deaths as low as possible. If it could be argued convincingly that some alternative allocation of the scarce resources probably would result in at least one more saved life, the contractors would agree to that alternative.[11]

In accepting both of the efficiency principles just discussed, the contractors would not be seeking to maximize goods other than the number of lives saved. They might know, for example, that the lives of some recipients would be potentially longer or more pleasant. But they would have no way of knowing which, if any, of these recipients they themselves might be. And, what is more important, since they would not know the details of their own life plans, they would be unable to judge their disvalue of, say, relative degrees of decreased function. What they would know is that life is essential to any life plan, and they would thus agree to measures that would preserve the best probability of sustaining life.

With their acceptance of these two efficiency principles, the contractors would have qualified the principle of equal access. No doubt they would consider similar principles should such be proposed. But it seems unlikely that they would limit equality of access for any but the most probable gains in efficiency. In other words, a basic presumption in favor of fair equality of access would remain. Appeals to efficiency would have to bear the burden of proof. In order to be acceptable, such appeals would have to give adequate reasons to expect a decrease in the probable number of deaths. This means that the principle of medical success, for example, would be interpreted rather generously. If there were uncertainties about a candidate's chances of medical success, it seems in keeping with the contractors' attitudes toward risk to say that they would favor erring, if necessary, on the side of including the candidate in the group to be given equal access.

Egalitarian Approaches and the Concept of Equal Access

Thus far, the deliberations of our hypothetical contractors concerning the distribution of scarce artificial hearts have led to the establishment of a presumption favoring the principle of fair equality of access. This principle has been qualified by an acceptance of efficiency principles only if they are likely to result in better chances of survival for a higher proportion of the potential recipients. Nothing, as yet, has been said about the procedural principles for instituting equal access. Nor has the concept of equal access been related to the various egalitarian approaches outlined in the last chapter. It is to these tasks that we now turn.

The principle of saving no one (E-1) would require little discussion by the deliberators. Even if the decision to "wait and die together" might sometimes be adjudged a courageous and noble act, from the perspective of the original position such sacrifice would always be considered a supererogation. Since the veil of ignorance assures impartiality, no accusation that the contractors developed principles to save themselves at the expense of others could be sustained.[12]

The principle of medical neediness (E-2) should also require only a brief discussion. The contractors would simply assume that all the potential recipients had essentially the same need for the resources; that is, without treatment the candidates would probably die, and with treatment they would probably live. Once this basic level of need had been established in some impartial way (that is, the levels of probability were applied evenhandedly), further gradients of medical neediness would matter little *unless* some efficiency principles were violated. For example, a candidate might need a high proportion of the available resources (for example, the services of medical personnel). In this sense, she or he could be said to have greater medical needs than other candidates. But these larger needs would not prevent equal access unless they ran counter to the principle of conservation. Similarly, greater medical need in terms of worse physical deterioration would not matter unless the probability of effective treatment fell below acceptable limits according to an impartially applied principle of medical success.

The principle of general neediness (E-3), which would give priority to those considered generally least well off, would be somewhat more troublesome and probably would require greater deliberation. At least initially, the principle would appear to be unattractive. This is so because of the incommensurability of life-saving health care with most other goods. If, as Rawls argues, the contractors would be unwilling to trade losses in liberty for gains in other goods, the same would be *a fortiori* true of trading off death-preventing medical resources. As Green remarks:

> Even more apparently than governmental interference, disease and ill health interfere with our happiness and undermine our self-confidence and self-respect. . . . [T]here seems to be little question that in the priorities or rational agents health care stands near to the basic liberties themselves.[13]

However, this issue becomes more difficult when stated in terms of whether or not the generally neediest should be granted priority as a means of redress. The questions of "restorative justice" are not easily addressed within a Rawlsian framework. Because of his emphasis on a "strict compliance" theory, Rawls says little about such problems as redress and retribution. These he considers elements of a "partial compliance" theory. And when, for example, Rawls does talk about a principle of redress he does not show how it might be derived from the original position.[14] He argues only that *some* of the objectives of redress can be achieved by adopting the difference principle. The difficulty of deriving principles of redress from Rawls's contract theory probably says more about an area in the theory needing development than about the unimportance of restorative justice.

A complete theory of social justice must include principles of compensation and redress. But attempting to state adequately how such principles might be derived from the perspective of contract theory would lead us astray at this point. With regard to triage, it seems unlikely that the contractors would agree to use a scarce resource such as the artificial heart as a means of compensating victims of unfair but relatively unrelated social practices. The reasons, again, would have to do with the incommensurability of life-saving resources with most other goods. However, at least intuitively, the case for "compensatory triage" would be stronger if the victims were suffering from some life-threatening malady because of injustices that had contributed to their general state of neediness as well as their medical neediness. Thus, a plausible argument might be made for giving victims of some unjust social activity (for example, poorly paid coal miners whose health and safety had been systematically ignored) priority in triage for a scarce new medical resource (for example, an artificial lung).

There are, to be sure, many complications with this approach. How probable must the case be for cause and effect? Would the victims have contracted the disease anyway? Are other medically needy candidates also victims? No doubt, in many instances such questions would be impossible to answer. But in spite of these and other difficulties, it is not unreasonable to think that contractors behind the veil of ignorance would agree to establish principles that would not only adequately protect them from being victimized by unjust social practices but also appropriately compensate them, even with medical resources, if such victimization should occur.

The final two egalitarian approaches discussed in the last chapter, queuing (E-4) and randomness (E-5), often have been viewed as roughly equivalent procedures for assuring equal access. But this equation deserves some scrutiny. As noted in the earlier discussion, the two practices may rest on rather different moral justifications.[15] What is more, it is not obvious that the two approaches would be equally effective in assuring fair equality of access.

145

Some who advocate the principle of queuing view it as a kind of "natural" random selection. Childress, for example, writes: "My proposal is that we use some form of randomness or chance (either natural, such as 'first come, first served,' or artificial, such as a lottery) to determine who shall be saved."[16] Thus, Childress considers both lottery and queuing to be means of securing equality of access. But later he makes it clear that he favors the "natural" approach of queuing because it "would be more feasible than a lottery since the applicants make their claims over a period of time rather than as a group at one time."[17] In his view, queuing has the distinct advantages of being in accordance with the way patients actually present themselves for treatment while at the same time affording the equal access of random selection.

But in order to say that the practice of "first come, first served" provides equal access it must be assumed (a) that the life-threatening disease is contracted more or less randomly, and (b) that the people who get the disease are able to enter and progress through the medical care system at roughly the same rate. Even if we leave aside questions about the first assumption, the second is sufficiently dubious to reduce confidence that queuing always assures equality of access. Human beings sometimes "jump the queue" even when what is desired is food in a cafeteria. If people's lives depend on their places in the queue, a policy of "first come, first served" would almost certainly result in a race for the scarce resources. And the most likely "winners" would not be the same as those selected randomly from the population in need. Those with sufficient means—wealth, power, information, contacts, confidence to enter the system, and so forth—would clearly have the competitive advantages. Though there are often no easy solutions to such problems, saying that queuing is the same as random selection ignores social and economic factors that may interfere with equal access. It is unlikely that contractors, knowing even the more general facts about human society, would prefer queuing as the primary means for instituting equality of access.

The "purer" way to guarantee equal access (disregarding certain objections for the moment) is some method of random selection or lottery. This is particularly obvious in a case such as that of the artificial heart, where it is likely that the needs of a large number of candidates throughout the society would *already* be known at least to some extent even before the technology becomes available. Under such circumstances, equality of access is more likely to be achieved if some truly random method of selection is instituted. Even though the context is far removed from a discussion of triage, Rawls makes essentially the same point when he says:

> [W]hen there are many equally strong claims which if taken together exceed what can be granted, some fair plan should be adopted so that all are equitably considered. In simple cases of claims to goods that are indivisible and fixed in number, some rotation or lottery scheme may be the fair solution when the number of equally valid claims is too great.[18]

Obviously the method of rotation would not be acceptable for the distribution of artificial hearts. But, even though there would undoubtedly be numerous difficulties, a lottery for the scarce devices would not be entirely impracticable, possibly even on a national scale. In fact, a kind of national medical triage using a lottery has at least one historical precedent. In 1953 the British Ministry of Health instituted a national lottery in order to allocate the scarce supplies of polio vaccine.[19] Birth dates were used as a basis for the random selection of eligible children. In many cases, families had some children who were selected and others who were not. But random selection was considered the fairest method for choosing the recipients.

A national lottery has also been proposed by Katz and Capron for the allocation of treatment for catastrophic diseases with scarce new technologies. In seeking an approach to decision making that would be "fair" and "rational," the authors suggest

> that treatment recipients can best be selected by a national system employing a mixture of collective standards and the lottery. In brief, such a system would rely on medical criteria to narrow the initial field of persons suffering from a catastrophic illness down to a pool of those who can reasonably be said to be likely to benefit from the treatment.

147

From this pool, regular drawings would be held whenever additional treatment spaces became available.[20]

There are good reasons to believe that this proposal is essentially similar to what contractors in the original position would unanimously accept. Provision is made for evaluations of medical suitability as measured by reasonable, impartially applied, and preferably public criteria. This part of the proposal is in accordance with the contract reasoning, set forth earlier, for the inclusion of principles of medical efficiency. The proposal also includes equality of access by random selection among the medically eligible candidates. Reliance on the lottery would appeal to the contractors not as a way of escaping moral responsibility or eliminating human judgments but rather as the fairest procedure for assuring equal access. At least since biblical times, the method of random selection has been adopted when two or more people have had equally strong (or weak) claims to some indivisible good.[21] No other procedure promises to be as impartial in the provision of equal access.

None of this means, of course, that a nationwide lottery for scarce medical resources would be trouble-free. Katz and Capron themselves recognize a number of potential difficulties. The magnitude of the national health care system, for example, would probably make the actual selections more feasible if conducted at the local or regional level. Nevertheless, the triage process still could be conducted under the aegis of national guidelines. The publicity of the decision making might also cause difficulties; the myth that society is willing to expend whatever means are necessary to save each and every life might be seriously eroded. On the other hand, to the extent that the myth of saving everyone is maintained, the publicity could lead to increased political pressures (as in the case of renal dialysis) to provide the treatment to all for whom it might be life-saving. Eventually, this pressure could lead to unbearable costs for increasingly elaborate medical care.

One further problem (one not mentioned by Katz and Capron) deserves attention. Any method of random selection has an unavoidable element of arbitrariness in its timing. This problem has both practical and theoretical ramifications. The lottery may provide equal access for candidates of known eligibility at the moment it is conducted. But, as Fried questions, why is that moment determinative?[22] The probability is high that waiting another day or week would allow additional candidates to be included in the selection process.

This problem of timing also raises related questions. Should subsequent lotteries include the names of all known candidates, or only the names of those who were not selected in earlier lotteries? Even though, as was argued earlier, a lottery and queuing are not the same, and even though equal access is better achieved by random selection, it is obvious that some elements of queuing would remain in any random selection system. This is true partly because of the need to set some time for the selection. The group from which the choices are made "got there first." Those who are still "on their way" are, in a sense, further back in the queue. Moreover, it is inconceivable that those who are selected first, and actually receive the scarce resources, would be placed again in subsequent selection pools. Once treatment had begun, legitimate expectations would be established, and no one would advocate having an artificial heart recipient enter each new lottery to see if the device should be retained or relinquished.

But, despite the various difficulties and necessary qualifications which have been recognized, the goal of providing fair equality of access to the scarce life-saving resources would remain the central concern of the rational contractors. And the most tenable method of achieving this goal would be random selection. The impossibility of instituting a lottery capable of perfectly achieving the goal does not invalidate the principle of equal access. The principle can still serve as a basis for criticizing the distribution system at all levels of its organization.

In sum, it has been argued in this section that rational deliberators behind the veil of ignorance would choose to allocate the kind of scarce medical resource represented by the artificial heart in accordance with a principle of fair equality of access. The contractors would not accept such utilitarian approaches as selection on the basis of general social worth. But they would incorporate in the triage process principles of efficiency that would maximize the probabilities of successful medical outcomes. Equality of access, instituted by a system of random

149

selection, would be for those candidates known to be medically eligible at the time of triage. Medical eligibility would be interpreted generously. But minimally it would require that there be reasonably good chances for medical success without using a disproportionately large amount of the resources. The presumption favoring equal access is complicated by the possibility of prior compensatory claims to the resources. But this possibility appears sufficiently remote so that it would be wiser to assume that the candidates all have equally strong claims to the resources and let claims to priority based on fair compensation bear the burden of proof. Fair equality of access is complicated further by the contingencies of queuing. Regardless of when the selections are made, the timing is bound to be somewhat arbitrary. In spite of this unavoidable arbitrariness, however, the timing of triage could only be called unjust if it effectively and systematically denied some class of potential candidates equal access to the scarce resources.

Has Rawls's device of the original position helped to bring greater coherence to our consideration of triage? Discussion of this question is postponed, for the most part, until the conclusion of this chapter. But some judgments are already obvious. Rawls's contractarian perspective focuses attention on human equality and the moral importance of impartiality. But the veil of ignorance does not eliminate all need for the balancing of utilitarian principles against strictly egalitarian principles. It is clear that Rawls's special conception of the principles of justice in their ranked order depends heavily on the ideal circumstances of his strict compliance theory. The further we move away from those ideal circumstances and into the "real world," the more other concerns, such as efficiency and coordination (whose importance Rawls also recognizes[23]), come to qualify principles such as fair equality of access. These qualifications are not imported into the list of principles after the contractors' deliberations. Rather, they stem directly from the kind of deliberations rational contractors would conduct, especially if the participants were primarily concerned about the worst possible outcomes. This same result may be seen again, perhaps more vividly, in the case of disaster triage.

Disaster Triage and the Difference Principle

The contract analysis of our other prismatic case, triage for a disaster, need not be as prolonged as the forgoing discussion of triage for the artificial heart. This is because many of the approaches to triage just discussed in connection with the artificial heart would receive similar judgments from the contractors. For example, the deliberators once again would agree to use the scarce resources in the most efficient ways in order to maximize the probability of saving the largest number of lives. The reasoning would be the same as before: the only way to guard against the worst outcome would be to reduce the probability of death due to lack of resources. Thus, the principle of medical success, which is often taken to be synonymous with the entire triage process in disaster situations, would be only one of the basic concerns, albeit an exceedingly important one. The principle of conservation also would be accepted by the contractors. Indeed, its appeal probably would be magnified by the emergent nature of the circumstances; large amounts of time or other resources which could be devoted to saving only one casualty might be used more efficiently to save the lives of several others.

There are other examples of approaches about which the decisions of the contractors would be essentially similar to those made about triage for the artificial heart. Again it would be assumed that all of the candidates had verified medical needs, although in the case of disaster triage the principle of medical neediness might be more readily superseded by the demands of efficiency. And once again the contractors would reject the broader utilitarian approaches, such as the principle of general social worth, not only because such principles would fail to appeal to the rational self-interest of the contractors but also because the contractors would know that such principles would be virtually impossible to apply.

But one of the more obvious differences in disaster triage would be the departure from equality of access in order to give priority to those most likely to benefit the community under

151

the immediate circumstances. Even those ethicists who vigorously advocate providing equality of access through the use of random selection generally recognize the need for a different approach in the unusual circumstances of disaster triage. For example, Ramsey says that "selecting patients by standards of worth to the group can be justified in only the exceptional case of communities of men who have (or have been reduced to) a focused social purpose."[24] But which focused social purposes are sufficient to override the presumption for equal consideration?

The one purpose that would have the most obvious appeal to rational contract agents would be lowering the probability of the worst possible outcome, in this case, death. The idea of giving priority to some casualties in order to aid others, which has been discussed earlier under the rubric of the principle of immediate usefulness, is akin to Rawls's difference principle. The favored treatment accorded to some would be acceptable to the contractors if, and only if, such a course could be reasonably expected to redound to the benefit of all, at least in terms of increased probabilities of being treated. On this principle, specially skilled persons, such as nurses, paramedics, physicians, and perhaps even police and fire personnel, could be given priority, insofar as it would be reasonable to expect their skills to be used for the benefit of other casualties. The appeal of this approach to the contractors is obvious. Whether the participants imagine themselves to be among the worst off casualties or among the ones given priority because of their immediate usefulness, this type of difference principle would appeal to both reason and self-interest.

In giving priority to those with special skills, the deliberators again would reveal the inevitability of some probabilistic thinking in the original position. Whether or not helping certain casualties actually would benefit others with greater needs, would, of course, always be open to some degree of uncertainty. Moreover, since some casualties still would be expected to die for want of medical attention, the benefits of favoring candidates with special abilities would not accrue to all in need. Indeed, there would always be the chance that the priority given to those who are believed to have special skills would actually be harmful to the worst off, who may die while waiting for the attention that could have been given to at least some of them instead of to the specially skilled ones. Obviously, the decision to favor the principle of immediate usefulness would hinge on probability calculations. But the contractors would be willing to do such calculations just because their attitude toward risk would lead them to minimize the probability of the worst possible outcome.

It is important, however, to distinguish the contract justification for the difference principle, which has been identified here with the principle of immediate usefulness, from a basically utilitarian rationale. It is not uncommon to find the principle of immediate usefulness understood simply in terms of the cost-benefit language of utilitarianism. For example, the author of one ethics textbook writes of the exceptional circumstances of the "the triage situation in medicine," and then makes the following comment:

> During a serious disaster when medical facilities simply cannot handle everyone who is injured, . . . an injured doctor or nurse who could be put to work would probably be the first to get medical attention since she or he would be able to save more of the other injured people than a nonmedical person. These, fortunately, are unusual circumstances which require different priorities from more normal situations. To apply the cost-benefit-analysis approach to the more normal situations, however, is tantamount to treating human beings as if they were some kind of inanimate 'product'.[25]

The author's point is to show that the utilitarian calculus which may be necessary in extreme situations, such as disaster triage, is not always appropriate when making more ordinary moral decisions.

But, as has already been seen, a difference principle, such as the principle of immediate usefulness, need not be justified simply in terms of a utilitarian calculus. Favoring the "doctor or nurse" may be viewed as a way of improving the prospects for the worst off. The difference principle, thus, represents an attempt to come as close as possible to equality of treatment in the long run,[26] and not just a means of maximizing utility. Although in practice the difference principle and an unembellished utilitarian approach may produce identical strategies, they clearly exemplify different perspectives.

153

In words which, in some ways, anticipated this part of Rawls's theory, Frankena reminds us of this distinction:

> [I]nequalities and differences in treatment are often said to be justified by their general utility. I do not deny this, but I do doubt that they can be shown to be *just* merely by an appeal to general utility. They can, however, often be shown to be just by an argument which is easily confused with that from the principle of utility: that initial inequalities in the distribution . . . are required for the promotion of equality in the long run.[27]

This is precisely the argument to appeal to the rational agents. Favoring those with special abilities would be a way of securing better odds on access to medical care for the worst off in the (not very) long run. Moreover, acceptance of the principle of immediate usefulness would qualify but not negate the prior presumption favoring equality of access. As was the case with other efficiency principles, this type of difference principle would have to bear the burden of proof. There would have to be ample reasons to believe that the special treatment given to some candidates would lead to benefits for the others, at least in terms of an increased probability of being given life-saving attention. Without such reasons, the principle of fair equality of access would stand. No doubt, the contingencies of disaster medicine would tend to limit severely the applicability of equal access, and the exception-making criteria of various efficiency principles would be met.

Equal access, in all likelihood, could only be implemented with the rough-and-ready method of treating casualties in the order of being found or brought to a treatment center. But, unlike triage for the artificial heart, the random nature of becoming a casualty, being rescued, and treated probably would be "lottery" enough to adequately approximate equality of access. Assuming that the casualties had neither special skills which would justify moving them ahead in the queue nor needs for disproportionately high amounts of the resources which would justify moving them back, the method of first come, first served among the medically eligible casualties would come as close as possible to equal access.

It is possible, of course, that a disaster, such as the next San Francisco earthquake, would be more devastating for some areas of the city than others (because of poor construction, for example). And it is not at all improbable that these harder-hit areas would be ones in which there would be fewer health care professionals and medical facilities. This would mean that the probability of being a casualty might be higher than the average and the probability of being treated might be lower in such areas. But in practical terms these problems could hardly be solved after the disaster in the immediate, microallocation situations. The deterrents to equal access probably would have to be removed through preplanning and macroallocation decisions (for example, in decisions about the location of facilities and in the planning for deployment of resources). Even though the present discussion has focused on the microallocation decisions, it is useful to mention the possibility of "built-in" hindrances to equality of access. We are thereby reminded that it may be virtually impossible to prescribe anything like a fair approach to triage without an awareness of the injustices endemic to the larger society.

Money and Merit

Some approaches to triage do not fit neatly in either the utilitarian or the egalitarian category. Two such bases for allocation, the ability to pay and past meritorious actions, were mentioned in passing in earlier chapters but deserve further comment before concluding. No ethicist has suggested that either money or merit should be the most important criteria for triage decision making. But both approaches have gained some prominence in the past, either because of proposed usage or because of actual usage in the selection of triage candidates.

The Ability to Pay

Although, so far as is known, dependence on the market system has never been made the *sole* method of distributing scarce life-saving medical resources, the ability of the triage candidate to pay for the treatment at times has been an important consideration in the decision making. For example, at one point during the earlier years of the Seattle Artificial Kidney Center, a patient's acceptance in the home dialysis program depended on his/her ability to pay an initial sum of $11,000 followed by payments of $250 per month.[28] If the in-center treatment slots were filled, and if the patient could not secure treatment at another center, the inability to pay for home dialysis presumably resulted in failure to obtain treatment, and, hence, death. And though deaths due to an inability to pay for treatment were probably rare, they were not unknown.[29]

But in spite of the fact that some candidates are likely to die for want of money, it has been argued that giving weight to a candidate's ability to pay is not only permissible but also better than some other alternatives. In favor of the market approach, it can be said that it is simpler and requires less intervention by authorities than various forms of collective decision making. Moreover, some commentators are convinced that triage based on the ability to pay, though imperfect, is at least more just than some other options.[30]

But is it possible that the "imperfections" of basing triage on the candidates' purchasing power could be ameliorated by adjustments in the market system? Katz and Capron suggest a number of modifications of the market that might make the market approach to triage more acceptable.[31] The authors argue that there are ways to structure the market other than simply permitting the scarce medical resources to go to the highest bidders. For example, each person in society could be given a right to an equal share of the scarce resources. People could then buy or sell shares as they saw fit. Risk-takers might sell their shares at a premium, while more cautious people might buy enough shares to assure receiving treatment if such became necessary. Another market system would depend on selling insurance policies to those who wished to protect themselves against some potentially life-threatening malady. But after considering some of the complications and difficulties with such proposals, the authors comment:

> [T]he market in catastrophic disease treatment would be less bothersome if we were confident that a man's wealth accurately reflected his worth to society, so the fact that a large percentage of rich people received the scarce lifesaving treatment could be said to result from their being more valuable. Yet such a premise would be dismissed out of hand by most people today, both as a factual matter and as a deviation from our collective ethic of equality of all persons.[32]

156

It *is* "our collective ethic," based on the fundamental principle of equal respect for persons, which precludes using the market system for triage. And if we once again allow the device of the original position to represent the "equality of all persons," it is not difficult to imagine the deliberations of the rational contractors. The contractors would not be willing to accept a selection system based on the candidates' ability to pay. Because of the veil of ignorance, they would not know whether they were rich or poor; thus they would not accept a principle that would give priority to the wealthy. They would know that any possible benefits to the poorer candidates, such as payment for shares purchased by the wealthier candidates, would be insufficient compensation for the loss of equal access to the scarce resources. Thus the contractors would agree with the conclusion of the Artificial Heart Assessment Panel:

> We believe that disparities in ability to pay which disparities hopefully will be eliminated through insurance or governmental measures—should not influence the decision, when implantation would appear to be beneficial, as to who will receive the artificial heart and who will be denied it.[33]

There remains, however, a special problem, which was raised briefly in chapter 4. Is it just to give priority to a wealthy candidate who promises to pay not only for his/her own treatment but also for the treatment of others? It will be remembered that the attorney on the patient selection committ in Seattle maintained that the answer to this question should be yes. And at least one writer has argued that an affirmative answer is prescribed by Rawls's theory. In a comment about scarce renal dialysis and the contract perspective, Freedman says that justice might require giving priority to those candidates who could be of some benefit to the others, and he adds:

> This would grant precedence to those who will donate money in full support of both their own dialysis and that of others. . . . Giving such individuals precedence would satisfy the 'difference principle' John Rawls included in his theory of justice.[34]

Favoring the wealthy candidate who promises to pay for the treatment of others does appear to be in harmony with Rawls's difference principle (or, to use our earlier designation, the principle of immediate usefulness). And it has been argued above that rational contractors would select this principle for triage situations in which it appeared reasonably certain that favoring one candidate would improve the chances of providing life-saving treatment for the others. Thus, to take an example from our earlier discussion, the nurse who, by hypothesis, must be treated before s/he can be of service to other disaster victims should be given priority.

It is obvious that the illustrations of the wealthy donor and the nurse are different in many ways. Some of these differences would appear to be morally relevant. The nurse *must* be treated first in order to benefit the other casualties. On the other hand, the wealthy candidate *could* contribute to the care of the others whether or not she or he is given priority. By using his or her wealth to secure favored treatment, the action of the rich candidate may be akin to a bribe. But neither this difference nor any others that come to mind would matter to the contractors. If accepting the rich candidate's offer would probably result in increased chances of treatment for the other candidates, it would be irrational for the contractors to reject the proposal.

If this outcome seems morally offensive, it is not so much the fault of the contract perspective as it is the error of viewing the specific case of the rich candidate in isolation from larger decisions about the health care system in general. In this study we have concentrated our attention on the microallocation decisions about scarce medical resources. But at times it is obviously impossible to ignore the broader questions about the organization of the health care system without attaining distorted results. So long as the affluent are able to buy more health care, including more life-saving health care, than the poor, it would be irrational for the contractors to decline the wealthy donor's bid for priority. But this does not mean that the contractors would approve of a market approach to the health care system in general. It is reasonable to think that the contractors would share with the Artificial Heart Assessment Panel the hope that disparities in levels of health care due to differences in the ability to pay will be eliminated from the larger system. The contractors would find the general system of health care based on the ability to pay at least as unacceptable as a market approach to the basic political liberties.

Rewarding Merit

Another approach to triage which does not fit the utilitarian/egalitarian schema is basing the selection on criteria of merit. Rescher calls this the "past-services-rendered factor." He contends that triage candidates who have given valuable services to the society may legitimately press their claims for just requital, including special priority in triage. As Rescher sees it: "It would be morally indefensible of society in effect to say: 'Never mind about services you rendered yesterday—it is only the services to be rendered tomorrow that will count with us today.'"[35]

The concept of just desert is exceedingly complex. It should be helpful to refer, even if briefly, to some of the entanglements, especially those that might have implications for triage.

First, the concept of merit should be distinguished from the utilitarian consideration of general social worth. As mentioned in chapter 4, merit generally refers to past action which leads to the approbation of *being worthy*. On the other hand, evaluations of a person's social value have to do with predictions of future contribution, or *having worth*.

Another difficulty with the concept of merit is the distinction between efforts and actual accomplishments. Should the reward go to those who expend great effort but with little success? Or should it be given to those who succeed with little or no effort? Or should both effort and success be required to establish a claim of just desert?

A third complication has to do with the distinction between moral and nonmoral merit. The notion that morally better people should reap more of society's rewards often has received support among moral philosophers. For example, in a well-known modern statement of this view, Ross argues that a "state of affairs in which the good are happy and the bad unhappy is better than one in which the good are unhappy and the bad happy."[36] According to Ross, distribution of the means of happiness in accordance with moral virtue is *the* duty of justice. In presenting this view, there can be little doubt that

159

Ross is in harmony with a widely held moral conviction: Virtuous people deserve better treatment. And, it might be added, there is no doubt that this view has sometimes affected triage decisions.[37]

But the kind of merit that has often given rise to the claim of just desert has not always had explicitly moral significance. Indeed, some have held that the qualities or actions considered to be the bases for good requital need not even be the result of the individual's choices.[38] It is clear that society often admires and rewards qualities regardless of the degree of volition. It is impossible to say, of course, just how much of the rationale for such rewards is actually utilitarian. But is seems clear that even without a utilitarian justification claims of just desert are often considered valid whether or not the merit required effort or choice. For example, graduate school admissions are granted not only on the basis of past scholastic performance (which presumably required some degree of will power and work) but also on the basis of test scores determined in large part by natural ability. In any case, it is generally impossible to tell where the gifts or accidents of nature and society terminate and the choices and efforts of the individual begin.

One final difficulty deserving mention is the relationship of merit to reward. Some rewards may be closely linked to the meritorious action (for example, when a student with good grades is awarded a scholarship). But in other instances, the type of reward may have no apparent relationship to the merit (for example, when a leading salesperson is awarded a trip to Hawaii). Rewards may be inappropriate in many ways. For example, the reward may be disproportionate (too large or too small) for the merit. But the appropriateness does not always depend on an obvious connection between the merit and the reward.

In spite of the complications just mentioned (and numerous others), there is a core to the concept of merit or just desert. Within a social context, an action or trait is judged to be admirable and some reward for that action or trait is judged to be appropriate. Or as Miller puts it:

> [D]esert is a matter of fitting forms of treatment to the
> specific qualities and actions of individuals, and in particular
> good desert . . . is a matter of fitting desired forms of treat-

ment to qualities and actions which are generally held in high regard.[39]

The question is this: What sort of merit, if any, could give rise to a decisive claim to scarce life-saving medical resources?

It is certain that the answer coming from the original position would be *none*. Contract theory generally plays down the importance of rewards for merit or for natural endowments. Indeed, this is one of the main reasons for selecting the contract perspective. Rawls says:

> Perhaps some will think that the person with greater natural endowments deserves those assets and the superior character that made their development possible. Because he is more worthy in this sense, he deserves the greater advantages that he could achieve with them. This view, however, is surely incorrect. It seems one of the fixed points of our considered judgments that no one deserves his place in the distribution of native endowments, any more than one deserves one's initial starting place in society.[40]

Thus, an important reason for adopting the contract view is that it "nullifies the accidents of natural endowment and the contingencies of social circumstance. . . ."[41]

Rawls admits there is a common-sense notion that, as a matter of justice, goods should be distributed in accordance with moral desert. But he says this view is flatly rejected in justice as fairness because "such a principle would not be chosen in the original position."[42] This does not mean that justice as fairness ignores all entitlements based on past actions. For example, rational contractors would agree to permit special rewards for those whose efforts or contributions ensure better conditions for everyone, especially the least advantaged. But such entitlements are the result of cooperation in a society already governed by just principles. Within a network of just social institutions, people develop legitimate expectations which entitle them to appropriate benefits. The principles of justice, on this view, do not automatically prescribe a distribution of rewards on the basis of merit. And there is no reason to think that the benefits will always match individual merit. Rather, the principles of justice chosen in the original position govern a "well-ordered" society within which legitimate expectations arise and entitlements are honored.

161

Needless to say, Rawls's treatment of merit has been one of the more disputed parts of the theory. Some critics have found Rawls's rejection of meritarian principles far too sweeping.[43] But whether any revision of contract theory could (or should) make more room for individual merit is not a question we need to consider here. So far as triage is concerned, the contractors' unwillingness to consider merit principles is certainly appropriate. A system of just institutions may foster the development of legitimate expectations in many ways. Thus a good student may be entitled to a better grade than a poor student, and a diligent worker may deserve a promotion before an indolent worker. But the first legitimate expectation with regard to health care is that those who are ill may expect equal access to the available medical resources. "Good people" are not entitled to more (or better) health care than "bad people." Health care is an inappropriate reward for meritorious action, either moral or nonmoral. This is true even when the merit in question has to do with taking proper care of one's own health.[44] One's place in the health/illness continuum may be influenced by too many imponderable factors, such as poor genetic endowment, irresponsible advertising, and an unhealthful work environment. Thus, it would be a mistake to allow even the merit of good personal health habits to influence decisions about those who deserve health care. To borrow a Rawlsian expression, one of the "fixed points" of our moral judgments is that health care, especially life-saving health care, is a social good to which all members of society are entitled simply on the basis of their medical needs. Without doubt, rational contractors would not agree to relinquish equal access to scarce medical resources in order to assure the distribution of those resources as rewards for merit.

Conclusion

The approaches to triage described in earlier chapters have now been "filtered" through Rawls's theory of justice. The result has not been a neat arrangement of all proposed triage principles in some ordinal ranking. Nor has the contract analysis eliminated all need for intuitive balancing of the various approaches. But such consequences are hardly surprising; the tragic circumstances of triage are far removed from Rawls's ideal theory with its special conception of just principles for the basic structure of society. Yet the contract perspective has not failed to structure our consideration of the various principles for triage. The deliberations of the contractors, it has been argued, would lead to the establishment of a presumption favoring fair equality of access to the scarce life-saving resources. Barring certain carefully defined exceptions, those who need the medical treatment in order to continue life would be granted equal consideration. Rational deliberators behind the veil of ignorance could not expect to get more, nor would they settle for less.

In relationship to this basic presumption favoring equality of access, the utilitarian and egalitarian principles outlined in the preceding chapters can be categorized in the following four ways: (1) constitutive principles, (2) provisory principles, (3) opposed principles, and (4) inappropriate principles. The constitutive principles are directly linked to the provision of fair equality of access. For example, the procedure of random selection is the most suitable way to assure equal access in some triage situations. In such cases, random selection is a necessary part of what it means to provide equal access. Provisory principles are understood as limitations on or qualifications of the presumption of equal access. The primary examples that would be accepted by the contractors would be the principles of conservation and medical success. And, in another way, some elements of queuing represent limitations on random selection of candidates for a scarce resource such as the artificial heart. The opposed principles are those that would be rejected from the perspective of justice as fairness. The principles of general social value and saving no one are examples. Finally, the inappropriate principles are those deemed inapplicable in the type of triage case under consideration. Such principles are not so much opposed to the selections of the contractors as they are simply inappropriate under the circumstances. Random selection in disaster triage and the principle of immediate usefulness in triage for the artificial heart are examples.

Table 2 is an attempt to represent the contractors' decisions about the various approaches to triage in terms of the four categories just defined.

TABLE 2
Decision Matrix For Triage Principles

Principle	Triage for TIAH				Triage for Disaster				Comments
	Constitutive	Provisory	Opposed	Inappropriate	Constitutive	Provisory	Opposed	Inappropriate	
U-1 Medical success		X				X			An efficiency limitation on equality of access selected for both cases in order to reduce the probability of wasted resources and thus reduce the probability of death due to lack of resources.
U-2 Immediate usefulness				X		X			Probably inapplicable for TIAH, but selected for disaster triage as a means of securing life-saving treatment for those whose lives are most endangered due to lack of such treatment.
U-3 Conservation		X				X			An important proviso selected for both cases so long as it could be reasonably demonstrated that at least one less life would probably be lost.
U-4 Parental role			X				X		The impartiality intended in the original position would lead to rejection of this principle, or so I have argued. In any event, the principle would certainly be inapplicable in disaster triage.
U-5 General social value			X				X		Unacceptable to the contractors because of their unwillingness to sacrifice equal access to the resources either for maximum general utility or to reward past merit.

				Comments
E-1 Saving no one		X	X	Considered either supererogatory or simply irrational, depending on the circumstances.
E-2 Medical neediness	X		X	An essential part of deciding which persons should be considered candidates. Assumed except for conflicts with provisory principles such as the principle of conservation.
E-3 General neediness		X	X	Generally considered inappropriate for triage because of an unwillingness to weigh life-saving resources in the same balance with other goods. Difficult to apply in microallocation circumstances.
E-4 Queuing	X	X		A partial but unavoidable limitation on the preferred procedure of random selection for TIAH. The only practical way to construe equal access in disaster triage.
E-5 Random selection	X		X	The chosen procedure for assuring equal access to TIAH, but inapplicable in disaster triage.

It may be objected that the decisions of the contractors have been reached at the expense of stretching Rawls's theory beyond acceptable limits. Without question, a discusion of triage fits uneasily in the framework of contract theory, and modifications of the theory have been necessary in order to accommodate the analysis of triage decision making.

Perhaps as significant as any of these alterations is the fact that the contractors have been allowed to take probability calculations into account more than Rawls appears to permit. The practical effect of such probabilistic reasoning is that the contractors would accept some principles of efficiency as limitations on equality of access. But, if the chances of the worst outcomes cannot be estimated in the way suggested in this chapter, it is doubtful that the deliberations could be called rational. The only way for the contractors to guard against the worst possible outcomes in triage is to reduce the probability that the scarce resources will be used so inefficiently that additional lives will be lost.

This necessity of probability calculations is not as inconsistent with Rawls's theory as it may at first appear. Even when the theory is not adjusted to the contingencies of triage, probabilistic reasoning would obviously be necessary to arrive at the selections Rawls attributes to the contractors. How else, for example, can the choice of the difference principle be understood? The contractors would surely have to know that for the difference principle to be applied, probability calculations would have to be done so that predictions about whether or not preferential treatment to person (or group) A might actually result in the greatest possible benefit to worst off person (or group) B. If, in answer, it is said that this assertion confuses the selection of basic principles by hypothetical contractors with the application of those principles by people outside the original position, then we may simply move the question back a step to the contract deliberations and ask: How, without some estimate of probabilities, could the contractors conclude that preferential treatment for some people in society would ever be likely to result in the highest minimum of any good for the worst off?

There is, of course, a danger in extending this line of reasoning too far. Rawls has attributed the characteristics of risk aversion and wariness of probability calculations to the contractors in order to avoid the counterintuitive selection of principles that would allow intolerable losses for a few in order to achieve some gain for the many. This is a legitimate concern and one not to be taken lightly, especially in designing the basic structure of an entire society. Nothing in the forgoing analysis denies this essential posture. But what is needed, at least in the case of triage, is a representation of the original position which allows limited kinds of probabilistic reasoning and yet guards against patently unjust selections. Such a construction is neither impossible nor inconsistent with the essential elements of Rawls's theory.

I conclude, then, by affirming that Rawls's conception of justice as fairness has assisted in the process of selecting, rejecting, and ordering the various approaches to triage. Aspects of the basic dilemma of conflicting utilitarian and egalitarian approaches obviously remain unresolved. But contract analysis has given definite structure to triage decision making by leading to the endorsement of a fundamental presumption in favor of the justness of equal access to the scarce life-saving medical resources. Exceptions to this basic principle have been limited in specific ways.

A Final Word

A sense of the tragedy of triage (and not just academic custom) prompts some final remarks of reservation. "The work of justice will be peace," the prophet says, "and the effect of justice, quietness and assurance forever."[45] But in this world our solutions are seldom, if ever, perfectly just. So our quietness and assurance are not everlasting; they are disturbed by intractable moral dilemmas. Michael Novak writes:

> Human communities of all kinds are, typically, not fair, and the exercise through which Rawls would put us is far too rational, procedural, and blind to the textures of human passion and quirk and contingency to help to express our actual grievances and hurts.[46]

True, the world is made neither of neat categories nor of fair people. This does not mean, however, that attempts to state

167

rational priciples of justice should cease, but that they should be tempered by humility and by frequent recourse to concrete historical experience. The problems of injustice may confound our best efforts, but we shall never know even how badly our efforts have been confounded unless we can gauge their distance from justice by some thoroughly considered principles.

Notes

I. The Concept of Triage in Modern Medicine

1. *Stedman's Medical Dictionary*, 22d ed. (Baltimore: William Wilkins Company, 1972), p. 1322.
2. *The Oxford English Dictionary*, Vol. XI: *T-U* (Oxford: Clarendon Press, 1933). Triage comes from the French *trier*, meaning "to pick" or "to cull." The word apparently entered English as a noun referring to the process of sorting agricultural products. Later it came to designate the lowest grade of such products—especially broken coffee beans.
3. See, for example, Stuart Hinds, "Triage in Medicine: A Personal History," in *Triage in Medicine and Society*, ed. George R. Lucas, Jr. (Houston: Institute of Religion and Human Development, 1975), pp. 8–9.
4. Robert G. Richardson, *Larrey: Surgeon to Napoleon's Imperial Guard* (London: John Murray, 1974), pp. 160–161.
5. Ibid., p. 34.
6. D. J. Larrey, *Surgical Memoirs of the Campaigns of Russia, Germany, and France*, trans. John C. Mercer (Philadelphia: Carey and Lea, 1832), p. 27.
7. Ibid., p. 109.
8. *The Surgical Memoirs of Baron Larrey*, Vols. I and II, trans. R. W. Hall; Vol. III, trans. J. C. Mercer (1812–1818), cited in Stuart Hinds, "On the Relations of Medical Triage to World Famine: An Historical Survey," in *Lifeboat Ethics: The Moral Dilemmas of World Hunger*, ed. George R. Lucas, Jr. and Thomas W. Ogletree (New York: Harper and Row, 1976), p. 32. [Emphasis added.]
9. Hinds, "Relations of Medical Triage to World Famine," p. 33.
10. These conditions are described in John Laffin, *Surgeons in the Field* (London: Aldine Press, 1970), pp. 156–157. The situation in the Union army at the beginning of the war was so dismal that a public uproar resulted. Reports of casualties being left unattended in the field for long periods of time led President Lincoln to establish a Sanitary Commission to aid the Medical Department

of the Army in caring for the sick and wounded. See also Harold Lueth, "Streamlining Military Medical Care," *Hygeia* XXI (March 1943): 194-195.

11. Walt Whitman, *The Wound Dresser: Letters Written to His Mother from the Hospitals in Washington During the Civil War,* ed. R. M. Bucke (New York: Bodley Press, 1949), p. 39.

12. Walt Whitman, *Complete Prose Works* (New York: Appleton and Company, 1910), p. 28.

13. John Hennen, *Principles of Military Surgery* (Philadelphia: Carey and Lea, 1830), pp. 64-70.

14. S. D. Gross, *A Manual of Military Surgery* (Philadelphia: J. B. Lippincott and Company, 1862), p. 31.

15. Ibid., p. 59.

16. Exceptions include the following: S. D. Gross, *A Manual of Military Surgery,* p. 44: "Dying patients should be carefully screened from their neighbors, placed in the easiest posture, have free access of air, and not be disturbed by noise, loud talking, or the presence of persons not needed for their comfort." L. Stromeyer, *Maximen der Kriegsheilkunst* (Hannover: Hahn'sche Hofbuchhandlung, 1855), p. 377: "Diejeniger, welche ihrem Ende nicht mehr fern sind, sollten von den übrigen so viel wie möglich getrennt und in den unteren Stockwerken untergebracht werden."

17. F. N. L. Poynter, ed., *Medicine and Surgery in the Great War (1914-1918)* (London: Wellcome Institute of the History of Medicine, 1968), introduction.

18. Laffin, *Surgeons in the Field,* p. 215. See also Kent Nelson, "An Army Motor Ambulance," *Military Surgeon* XXXVIII (February, 1916): 151-167. In this article Nelson shows that a mule-drawn ambulance cost $1 more to put in the field than a Ford motorized ambulance ($1147 to $1146). Near the end of the war authors were still calling for more motorized ambulances. See, for example, Percy Jones, "Motor Ambulance and Personnel," *Military Surgeon* XL (May, 1917): 572-574.

19. W. W. Keen, *The Treatment of War Wounds* (Philadelphia: W. B. Saunders Company, 1917), p. 13. [Emphasis added.]

20. Both the term "triage" and the idea of a sorting station were new to the American army in World War I, having been borrowed from the French and British allies. Frank W. Weed, *Field Operations,* Vol. VIII: *The Medical Department of the United States Army in the World War* (Washington, D.C.: United States Government Printing Office, 1925), p. 143. In a "glossary of French expressions," another work contains the following entry: "Triage: sorting station; the act of sorting; or the field hospital where the wounded are sorted and directed to various base hospitals in the vicinity according to the nature of their wounds or illness and the treatment required." *History of the American Field Service in France,* Vol. III (Boston: Houghton Mifflin Company, 1920).

21. For an example of such a diagram see W. S. Bainbridge, *Report on Medical and Surgical Developments of the War* (Washington, D.C.: United States Government Printing Office, 1919), p. 217.
22. Adapted from Paul F. Straub, *Medical Service in Campaign: A Handbook for Medical Officers in the Field* (Philadelphia: P. Blakiston's Son and Company, 1910), pp. 47 ff. Even though this work was published prior to World War I, its categories for casualty sorting and the underlying reasoning are indicative of the developments taking place during this time. For example, the book states: "It is gradually becoming more and more appreciated that the care and treatment of the less severe cases is of greater importance to the army in the field than that of the serious ones. . . . " p. 48.
23. Adapted from John McCombe, and A. F. Menzies, *Medical Service at the Front* (Philadelphia: Lea and Febiger, 1918), pp. 124–125. Numerous additional triage plans could be listed. See, for example, Weed, *Field Operations*, pp. 143 ff. and Cuthbert Wallace and John Fraser, *Surgery at a Casualty Clearing Station* (London: A. and C. Black, 1918), p. 4.
24. Laffin, *Surgeons in the Field*, p. 233.
25. G. W. Crile, "Summarized Report of the Conference on Surgery in Battle Areas," *War Medicine* (October 1918): 298.
26. See, for example, Roger I. Lee, "The Case for the More Efficient Treatment of Light Casualties in Military Hospitals," *Military Surgeon* XLII (March 1918): 283–285.
27. A. D. Tuttle, *Handbook for the Medical Soldier* (New York: William Wood and Company, 1927), pp. 84–85.
28. *"The Tale of a Casualty Clearing Station,"* Blackwood's Edinburgh Magazine CC (November 1916): 637.
29. Probably the most often-cited triage plan is in Jose Trueta, *Principles and Practice of War Surgery* (St. Louis: C. V. Mosby Company, 1943), pp. 178 ff.
30. These figures are taken from the compilation in Gilbert W. Beebe and Michael E. DeBakey, *Battle Casualties: Incidence, Mortality, and Logistic Considerations* (Springfield, Ill.: Charles C. Thomas, 1952), p. 77.
31. Chester Keefer, "Penicillin: A Wartime Achievement," in *Advances in Military Medicine*, Vol. II, ed. E. C. Andrus et al. (Boston: Little, Brown and Company, 1948), pp. 717–722.
32. Ibid., p. 719.
33. Henry K. Beecher, "Scarce Resources and Medical Advancement," in *Experimentation with Human Subjects*, ed. Paul A. Freund (New York: George Braziller, 1969), pp. 66–104.
34. Hinds, "Triage in Medicine," p. 12.
35. Beebe and DeBakey, *Battle Casualties*, p. 5.
36. *Emergency War Surgery* (Washington, D.C.: United States Government Printing Office, 1958), p. 168. This is the United States armed forces issue of the NATO handbook.

37. Ibid., p. 33. [Emphasis added.]
38. Hinds, "Relations of Medical Triage to World Famine," p. 46. In fairness, it must be mentioned that Hinds's main point is to show the inappropriateness of the concepts and language of medical triage to the discussions of world famine. Nevertheless, he builds his argument to a large extent on the contention that triage in military medicine was always based on the medical needs of the casualties. But even Hinds's own illustrations tend to refute this contention.
39. Beebe and DeBakey, *Battle Casualties*, p. 216 [emphasis added]. The use of medicine for the sake of military victory has led some critics to conclude that the morality of medicine is completely compromised in the military setting. For example, Livingston writes: "[I]t seems clear to me that to the degree that the needs of the military are inherently inimical to the needs of those whom it uses, the physician who must deal with both is confronted with a divided loyalty, and the pressure to conform to the needs of the organization is nearly irresistible." Gordon S. Livingston, "Medicine and the Military," in *Humanistic Perspectives in Medical Ethics*, ed. Maurice B. Visscher (Buffalo: Prometheus Books, 1972), pp. 266–274. See also Perry London and H. Tristram Engelhardt, Jr., "Fear of Flying: The Psychiatrist's Role in War," *Hastings Center Report* VI (February, 1976): 20–21. These two authors take up the issue of whether the military doctor's loyalties should be to the soldiers or to the state.
40. H. Tristram Engelhardt, Jr., "Individuals and Communities, Present and Future: Towards a Morality in a Time of Famine," in *Lifeboat Ethics: The Moral Dilemmas of World Hunger*, ed. George R. Lucas, Jr. and Thomas W. Ogletree (New York: Harper and Row, 1976), p. 82.
41. See, for example, J. F. Fulton, "Medicine, Warfare, and History," *Journal of the American Medical Association* CLIII (October 3, 1953): 482–488.
42. In one survey, when physicians were asked about their training in the sorting and care of mass casualties, 74 percent indicated they had been trained in military service. Donald P. Dressler et al., "The Physician and Mass Casualty Care: A Survey of Massachusetts Physicians," *Journal of Trauma* XI (March, 1971): 260–262.
43. See, for example, Eugene D. Gierson and Leon S. Richman, "Valley Triage: An Approach to Mass Casualty Care," *Journal of Trauma* XV (March, 1975): 193–196.
44. See, for example, Donald M. Vickery, *Triage: Problem-Oriented Sorting of Patients* (Bowie, Maryland: Robert J. Brady, 1975): Kathryn A. McLeod, "Learning to Take the Trauma of Triage," *RN* XXXVIII (July, 1975): 23–27; Peter Rosen et al., "A Method of Triage within an Emergency Department," *JACEP* III (March/April, 1974): 85, 86.

45. The expression "high technologies" as applied to medicine has become relatively common usage, albeit generally ill defined. The phrase usually refers to new and costly treatments, which one author has called "halfway technology." See Lewis Thomas, "Guessing and Knowing: Reflections on the Science and Technology of Medicine," *Saturday Review* 23 December 1972, pp. 52–57.

46. For a comprehensive and careful account of the patient selection process developed in the early years of the Seattle Artificial Kidney Center, see Renee C. Fox and Judith P. Swazey, *The Courage to Fail* (Chicago: University of Chicago Press, 1974), pp. 215–316. See also Richard A. Rettig, *Health Care Technology: Lessons Learned from the End-Stage Renal Disease Experience* (Santa Monica: Rand Corporation, 1976).

47. Scribner's personal account of his discovery is in Gary Cavalli, "Imagination, Work, and the Arteriovenous Shunt," *Stanford M.D.* XIII (Summer 1974): 2.

48. Some of Scribner's first patients were still alive in the 1970s, more than ten years after their first dialyses. See Fox and Swazey, *Courage to Fail*, p. 222.

49. These figures are taken from "Scarce Medical Resources," *Columbia Law Review* LXIX (April 1969): 637. For more recent cost estimates see Deborah Shapley, "National Health Insurance: Will It Promote Costly Technology?" *Science* CLXXXVI (November, 1974): 425; and Carol Levine, "Home Dialysis and the Medicare Gap," *Hastings Center Report* VI (December 1976): 5–6. In this article the author indicates that home dialysis costs from $6000 to $8000 per year, and in-center dialysis ranges from $24,000 to $30,000 per year. See also Willem J. Kolff, "Cost and Technology: Artificial Kidneys," *Clinical Engineering* 7 (January-February, 1979): 10.

50. For an explanation of the purpose of the committee from the perspective of the medical personnel who were instrumental in initiating the idea, see J. Murray et al., "A Community Hemodialysis Center for the Treatment of Chronic Uremia," *Transactions of the American Society for Artificial Internal Organs* VIII (1962): 315–319.

51. Fox and Swazey, *Courage to Fail*, p. 245.

52. Shana Alexander, "They Decide Who Lives, Who Dies: Medical Miracle Puts a Moral Burden on a Small Committee," *Life* 9 November 1962, pp. 102 ff.

53. In the case of the children the decision was based on the fact that they would not be able to mature normally because hemodialysis inhibits the onset of puberty. The reason for the upper age limit is less clear. Presumably older patients are more susceptible to medical complications. But as dialysis developed in the 1960s, vastly different age limits were set in various artificial kidney centers. One clinic, for example, had limits below the age of five

or over sixty. For a discussion of age as a criterion of exclusion see "Scarce Medical Resources," pp. 644–645.

54. Alexander, "They Decide," p. 115.
55. Ibid.
56. Ibid., p. 123.
57. Ibid., p. 115.
58. Ibid., p. 117.
59. Ibid., p. 118.
60. Ibid., p. 106.
61. David Sanders and Jesse Dukeminier, Jr., "Medical Advance and Legal Lag: Hemodialysis and Kidney Transplantation," *U.C.L.A. Law Review* XV (February 1968): 378.
62. Alexander, "They Decide," p. 123.
63. Sanders and Dukeminier, "Medical Advance," p. 378.
64. A. H. Katz and D. M. Procter, *Social-psychological Characteristics of Patients Receiving Hemodialysis Treatment for Chronic Renal Failure*, mimeographed (Washington D.C.: Department of Health, Education, and Welfare, July 1969).
65. Fox and Swazey, *Courage to Fail*, p. 244.
66. Leo Shatin, "Medical Care and the Social Worth of Man," *American Journal of Orthopsychiatry* XXXVI (1966): 96–101.
67. Ibid., p. 97.
68. Ibid., p. 99.
69. G. E. Schreiner, "Problems of Ethics in Relation to Haemodialysis and Transplantation," in *Ethics in Medical Progress*, ed. G. E. W. Wolstenholme (Boston: Little, Brown and Company, 1966), p. 128.
70. Ibid., p. 127.
71. In addition to the study by Katz and Procter, see "Scarce Medical Resources," pp. 639–662. The researchers who compiled data for this law journal article conducted extensive telephone interviews with many of the leading artificial kidney centers.
72. Katz and Procter, *Characteristics of Patients Receiving Hemodialysis*, p. 23.
73. See, for example, Lawrence K. Altman, "Artificial Kidney Use Poses Awesome Questions," *New York Times* 24 October 1971, pp. 1, 49; J. Hyatt, "The Cost of Living: Some Kidney Patients Die for Lack of Funds for Machine Treatment," *Wall Street Journal* 10 March 1969, p. 1, 19.
74. Fox and Swazey, *Courage to Fail*, p. 249.
75. Eli A. Friedman and Samuel Kountz, "Impact of HR-1 on the Therapy of End-Stage Uremia," *New England Journal of Medicine* CCLXXXVIII (14 June 1973): 1286–1288.
76. See, for example, Gordon L. Moore, "Who Should Be Dialyzed," *American Journal of Psychiatry* CXXVII (March 1971): 1208–1209.
77. For an example of this usage see "Scarce Medical Resources," pp. 635 ff and 670 ff.

78. From Dr. Belding Scribner's testimony before the House Ways and Means Committee, 25 April 1977, as reported by Associated Press International, 26 April 1977. For a discussion of many of the problems still facing renal dialysis patients see Gerald Perkoff et al., "Long Term Dialysis Programs: New Selection Criteria, New Problems," *Hastings Center Report* VI (June 1976): 8-13.
79. Alexander, "They Decide," p. 124.
80. "A Life in the Balance," *Time*, 3 November 1975, p. 61. The language and categories of triage have begun to appear in the context of discussions of world hunger, far removed from medicine. Perhaps the best-known early usage is William Paddock and Paul Paddock "Herewith Is a Proposal for the Use of American Food: 'Triage,'" in *Famine—1975!* (Boston: Little, Brown, and Company, 1967), chap. 5. See also Wade Green, "Triage," *New York Times Magazine*, 5 January 1975, pp. 111-122.
81. Richard Titmuss, *The Gift Relation* (New York: Vintage Books, 1971), pp. 64-66.
82. Rosemary Biggs, "Supply of Blood-Clotting-Factor VIII for Treatment of Haemophilia," *Lancet* I (29 June 1974): 1339. The author indicates that a chronic shortage of blood-clotting factor in Great Britain has led to undertreatment with increased morbidity and mortality. The primary reason for the shortage is lack of money.
83. L. Brent, ed., "The Shortage of Organs for Clinical Transplantation: Document for Discussion," *British Medical Journal*, I (February, 1975): 251-255. The shortage of available kidneys in the U.S. has even prompted some people to advertise one of their kidneys for sale. See "Body Parts for Sale," *Hastings Center Report* VI (February 1976): 2.
84. A. Earl Walker, "The Neurosurgeon's Responsibility for Organ Procurement," *Journal of Neurosurgery* XLIV (January 1976): 1-2.
85. See, for example, Harry Schwartz, "Must Doctors Serve Where They're Told?" *New York Times*, 14 March 1976, p. 16. According to this report, the number of physicians per 100,000 people in the United States ranged from 265 in California to 87 in South Dakota.
86. Chayet has raised questions from a *legal* perspective about the practice of medical triage in disaster situations. Among other problems, Chayet claims that the physician who practices triage may be guilty of abandonment under present legal codes. But his main concern seems to be the threat of a lawsuit for the physician. He writes with acerbity: "[I]t would appear that in most states the physician has two choices: he must either make a lawyer a part of the triage team, or he must completely ignore the disaster legislation as presently constituted." Neil L. Chayet, *Legal Implications of Emergency Care* (New York: Appleton-Century-Crofts, 1969), p. 126.
87. An exception is Thomas O'Donnell, "The Morality of Triage," *Georgetown Medical Bulletin* XIV (August 1960): 68-71.

II. Two Prismatic Cases

1. I have borrowed this expression from Edmond Cahn, *The Moral Decision: Right and Wrong in the Light of American Law* (Bloomington: Indiana University Press, 1955), p. 245.
2. When the research for this chapter was initiated, the director of San Francisco's Office of Emergency Services was Edward P. Joyce. The present director is Philip S. Day, Jr.
3. Ted Morgan, "The Good Life (Along the San Andreas Fault)," *New York Times Magazine*, 4 July 1976, p. 18.
4. Office of Emergency Services, City and County of San Francisco, "San Francisco Earthquake Response Plan," mimeographed (San Francisco: September, 1974), chart no. 2. It should be noted that these estimates are for the nine counties of the Bay Area.
5. Ibid., chart no. 3. For example, an estimated 50,000 lives would be lost in the event of the failure of just one dam.
6. Donald Trunkey, private interview, San Francisco, 17 February 1977. Formerly in charge of the San Francisco Medical Association's emergency planning, Dr. Trunkey is on the staff of the San Francisco General Hospital.
7. Office of Emergency Services, City and County of San Francisco, "Emergency Medical Care: General Operational Procedures," mimeographed (San Francisco: March 1976), p. 11.
8. "Earthquake Response Plan," p. A-4.
9. These zones and the various emergency facilities within the ten districts in the main part of the city are outlined in "Emergency Medical Care." See also Verne Paule, "San Francisco Gets Ready," *Foresight* (March-April 1975), pp. 24–29. The overall plan is further outlined in Office of Emergency Services, City and County of San Francisco, "Medical and Health Annex: Emergency Operations Plan," mimeographed (San Francisco: March 1976). This plan is currently being rewritten. Philip S. Day, Jr., personal letter, 31 July 1980.
10. "Earthquake Response Plan," p. 2.
11. "Emergency Operations Plan," p. 4.
12. Edward P. Joyce, private interview, 2 August 1976.
13. "Emergency Operations Plan," p. 3.
14. Joyce interview.
15. "Earthquake Response Plan," p. 4.
16. "The Place of Biomedical Science in Medicine and the State of Science," Appendix A of *Report of the President's Biomedical Research Panel* (Washington, D.C.: United States Government Printing Office, 1976) [Department of Health, Education, and Welfare Publication No. (OS)76–501].
17. Ibid., p. 219.
18. Two of TIAH's main developers have written: "The artificial heart is almost ready for clinical application." W. J. Kolff and J.

Lawson, "Perspectives for the Total Artificial Heart," *Transplantation Proceedings* 11 (March 1979): 317. See also "Mechanically Assisted Circulation—The Status of the NHLBI Program and Recommendations for the Future," *Artificial Organs* 1 (November 1977): 39–58.

19. Ibid.

20. Most of these remarks on the history of the artificial heart are based on information given in *The Totally Implantable Artificial Heart: Economic, Ethical, Legal, Medical, Psychiatric, Social Implications* (Washington, D.C.: Department of Health, Education, and Welfare, 1973), pp. 17–19 and 203–214 (hereinafter referred to as *Artificial Heart*). See also George B. Griffenhagen and Calvin H. Hughes, "The History of the Mechanical Heart," *Annual Report of the Smithsonian Institution, 1955* (Washington, D.C.: United States Government Printing Office, 1956), pp. 339–352.

21. It is interesting to note that already in 1955 a professional society for medical researchers interested in the development of artificial organs, the American Society for Artificial Internal Organs, was being established. For a short history of the society, see G. E. Schreiner, "Introduction," *Transactions: American Society for Artificial Internal Organs* XXII (1976): xvii.

22. According to Harvey M. Sapolsky, the annual expenditure has been about eight to ten million dollars. "Government and the Development of the Artificial Heart," in *Artificial Heart*, Appendix A, p. 213. This level of funding has remained fairly constant to the present time. It should be noted, however, that the *percentage* of NHLI's budget for heart research earmarked for TIAH has been gradually dropping.

23. For an article that describes German research, see U. Nemsmann, "Driving Systems for Artificial Blood Pumps," *Transactions: American Society for Artificial Internal Organs* XXII (1976): 128–134.

24. "Detente and the Artificial Heart," *Science Digest* LXXX (November 1976): 14–15.

25. For an explanation of some of the technical problems, see D. H. Rimbey, "Magnetic Heart Pump Challenge," *Mechanical Engineering* XCVII (June 1976): 36–38.

26. "Rubber Research on Artificial Heart Progresses," *Chemical and Engineering News* LIV (17 May 1976): 24–26.

27. *Report of the President's Biomedical Research Panel*, Appendix A, p. 219.

28. See, for example, John Lawson and Willem J. Kolff, "The Artificial Heart: Current Status and Clinical Prospects," *Practical Cardiology* 5 (July 1979): 95–103.

29. Kolff and Lawson, "Perspectives for the Total Artificial Heart," p. 319.

30. Belding Scribner, private interview, quoted in Renee C. Fox and

Judith P. Swazey, *The Courage to Fail*, (Chicago: University of Chicago Press, 1974), p. 329.

31. The panel members were: Alfred P. Fishman, Harold P. Green, Herbert E. Griswold, Jr., Clark C. Havighurst, Albert R. Jonsen, Norman Kaplan, Jay Katz, Harvey M. Sapolsky, David S. Salkever, and Mabel M. Smythe.
32. For a full statement of the panel's charge, see *Artificial Heart*, p. 14.
33. Ibid., p. xiv.
34. Ibid., p. 187.
35. Ibid., p. 190.
36. Ibid., p. 115. For example, it was estimated that the use of nuclear power sources in a fully implemented program of artificial heart implantation might result in one excess case of cancer per 7,200 spontaneous cases.
37. Ibid., p. 61.
38. Ibid.
39. It is interesting to note that (according to one report) two of the panel members had read Rawls's *A Theory of Justice* just prior to the panel's meetings. Morris Bernard Kaplan, "The Case of the Artificial Heart Panel," *Hastings Center Report* V (October 1975): 47.
40. *Artificial Heart*, p. 72. The low-end estimates were $15,000 and 16,750 participants.
41. Ibid.
42. Ibid., p. 142.
43. Ibid., p. 148.
44. Ibid., p. 147.
45. Ibid.
46. Ibid., p. 231.
47. Ibid., p. 233.
48. Ibid., p. 245.
49. Ibid., pp. 10–11. Professor Kaplan dissociated himself from this portion of the panel's report.
50. Ibid., p. 244.
51. For a helpful discussion of statistical lives as opposed to identifiable lives, see generally Guido Calabresi and Philip Bobbitt, *Tragic Choices* (New York: W. W. Norton, 1978).
52. Albert R. Jonsen, "The Totally Implantable Artificial Heart," *Hastings Center Report* V (November 1973): 4.
53. Martin Koughan, "Goodbye, San Francisco: Measuring the Effect of the Inevitable Earthquake," *Harper's Magazine*, September 1974, p. 32.
54. *Report of the President's Biomedical Research Panel*, p. 219.
55. W. J. Kolff, *Artificial Organs* (New York: John Wiley and Sons, 1976), pp. 52–59. This work also includes extensive bibliographies and many useful illustrations.

III. Dire Scarcity and Distributive Justice

1. Nicholas Rescher, *Distributive Justice: A Constructive Critique of the Utilitarian Theory of Distribution* (New York: Bobbs-Merrill Company, 1966), p. 96.
2. Lewis Thomas, "Guessing and Knowing: Reflections on the Science and Technology of Medicine," *Saturday Review*, 23 December 1972, p. 56. Thomas advocates concentrating money and efforts on finding cures for diseases rather than on expensive technologies to ameliorate the course of disease. For the arguments of one who says that it would be immoral to give priority to the prevention and cure of disease rather than to the medical care of those who are already ill, see Benjamin Freedman, "The Case for Medical Care, Inefficient or Not," *Hastings Center Report* VII (April 1977): 31–39.
3. Abraham Maslow, *Motivation and Personality* (New York: Harper and Row, 1954).
4. John Rawls, *A Theory of Justice* (Cambridge: Harvard University Press, 1971), p. 92.
5. For a discussion of the concept of "false needs" see H. Marcuse, *One-Dimensional Man* (Boston: Beacon, 1964).
6. Brian Barry, *Political Argument* (London: Routledge and Kegan Paul, 1965), Chapter III.
7. I have taken this argument from David Miller, *Social Justice* (Oxford: Clarendon Press, 1976), pp. 130 ff. There are, of course, other ways in which a need might be deemed "false."
8. It would be impossible, for example, for the patient to make the final decision if s/he were unconscious and if the decision could not be postponed. For a discussion of this problem see Karen Tait and Gerald Winslow, "Beyond Consent—The Ethics of Decision-Making in Emergency Medicine," *Western Journal of Medicine* CXXVI (February 1977): 156–159.
9. *The Totally Implantable Artificial Heart: Economic, Ethical, Legal, Medical, Psychiatric, Social Implications* (Washington, D.C.: Department of Health, Education, and Welfare, 1973), p. 66 (hereinafter referred to as *Artificial Heart*), p. 66.
10. Grant Fjermedal, "Growth Hormone Determines Stature," *Science News Service*, 18 May 1977. It should be noted that this article was written prior to the application of recombinant DNA techniques to the production of growth hormone. There is now hope that the new technology will eliminate scarcities of the hormone.
11. Nicholas Rescher uses a similar expression for a somewhat different meaning. *Distributive Justice*, p. 97.
12. See, for example, Robert T. Garner and Bernard Rosen, *Moral*

Philosophy: A Systematic Introduction to Normative Ethics and Metaethics (New York: Macmillan Company, 1967), pp. 185 ff.

13. Vivian Charles Walsh, *Scarcity and Evil* (Englewood Cliffs: Prentice-Hall, 1961), p. 71.

14. Ibid., p. 8.

15. Dr. Hunt's comments are found in A. R. Jonsen et al., "Critical Issues in Newborn Intensive Care: A Conference Report and Policy Proposal," *Pediatrics* LV (June 1975): 763. The authors of this report stated the following principle for neonatal triage: "[G]iven the impossibility of treating all infants in need, those should have preference who give the greatest hope of surviving with maximal function." But the authors went on to list several cautions about the use of this principle, and they concluded that "the principle of neonatal triage, while instructive in general, is fraught with the risk of serious bias."

16. Rawls, for example, says that his position concerning the circumstances of justice "largely follows that of Hume." *Theory of Justice*, p. 126. Most of Hume's thoughts on justice are recorded in two places: *A Treatise of Human Nature*, Book III, Part II, and *An Enquiry Concerning the Principles of Morals*, section III. For an extensive analysis of Hume's arguments concerning the conditions of justice, see D. Clayton Hubin, "The Scope of Justice," *Philosophy and Public Affairs* 9 (Fall 1979): 3–24.

17. David Hume, *An Enquiry Concerning the Principles of Morals*, Section III, Part I, in *Enquiries Concerning Human Understanding and Concerning the Principles of Morals*, ed. L. A. Selby-Bigge (Oxford: Clarendon Press, 1975), p. 183. (hereinafter cited as *Enquiry*).

18. Ibid., p. 184.

19. "Competition" is used here in a restricted sense. Hume does not envision a society in which people climb ladders of success, wealth, and power. He is more interested in having people be content with their stations in existing society. Thus, Miller is correct in saying that "Hume did not see society as the utilitarian economists did, as the interplay of competitive, egoistic individuals, held together by the bonds of mutual interest." David Miller, *Social Justice*, p. 178. Hume does not mention competition per se, nor does he stress self-interest in the way some of the later utilitarians did. But as Miller also recognizes and, as will be emphasized more below, Hume does perceive society to be marked by some conflict of interests which the rules of justice are intended to settle.

20. Hume, *Enquiry*, p. 186.

21. Ibid.

22. See, for example, C. D. Broad, *Five Types of Ethical Theory* (London: Routledge and Kegan Paul, 1930), Chapter IV.

23. David Hume, *A Treatise of Human Nature*, Part II, Section II, in Hume's Ethical Writings, ed. Alasdair MacIntyre (London:

Collier-Macmillan, 1965), pp. 221–222. (hereinafter cited as *Treatise*).

24. Ibid.
25. Rawls, *Theory of Justice*, p. 32.
26. Hume, *Enquiry*, p. 187.
27. See David Hume, *Of the Original Contract* in *Hume's Ethical Writings*, ed. Alasdair MacIntyre, p. 255 ff.
28. For his discussion of "natural" and "artificial" see *Enquiry*, pp. 307 ff. In saying that justice is an "artificial" virtue, Hume means that it is not one of the spontaneous reactions of human emotions but rather requires reason, forethought, and planning.
29. Some empirical studies have shown that people react to disaster with far more order and less panic than might be expected. In studies of over 100 disasters, researchers at Ohio State University's Disaster Research Center found that panic almost never occurs during or after a disaster. The vast majority of people respond by giving mutual aid, supporting the efforts of authorities, and rescuing the trapped and injured. Indeed, one of the unexpected consequences of most disasters is the *heightened* morale within the communities. The report concluded: "The reality suggests that human beings are amazingly resilient in the face of adversity. Perhaps heroism is not the wrong word to describe disaster behavior." E. L. Quarantelli and R. Dynes, "When Disaster Strikes," *Psychology Today*, February 1972, pp. 67–70. See also Katherine Byrn, "Disaster Brings Out the Best in People," *Science Digest*, August 1973, pp. 29–34.

    However, the effects of long-term adversities, such as scarcities of needed resources, may be devastating to a community. In his classic study, Sorokin shows how scarcity can lead to the breakdown of society as practices such as stealing, prostitution, and even cannibalism become prevalent. Pitirim A. Sorokin, *Man and Society in Calamity* (New York: E. P. Dutton, 1942). In a more recent study which tends to confirm Sorokin's conclusion, anthropologist Colin Turnbull describes the plight of the Ik people of East Africa. The Ik lost their traditional hunting grounds because of the creation of a national game reserve. Unable to adjust to farming in an arid and infertile land, the once prosperous Ik were reduced to extreme poverty and starvation with devastating effects on the community. According to Turnbull, all vestiges of human concern and compassion, even within families, gave way to self-interested striving for survival. Colin M. Turnbull, *The Mountain People* (New York: Simon and Schuster, 1972).
30. It should be mentioned that the legality of commandeering the services of medical personnel is uncertain. Chayet says: "In most states . . . the governor cannot seize the services of individuals such as physicians." Neil Chayet, *Legal Implications of Emergency Care* (New York: Appleton-Century-Crofts, 1969), p. 117. But Chayet says that Washington state is an exception, and he raises

questions about the status of medical personnel at government-owned institutions.

31. *Artificial Heart*, p. 198.
32. For an extensive treatment of the relationship between Hume's vision of society and his theory of justice see David Miller's chapter, "Hume's Theory of Justice," in *Social Justice*, pp. 157–179.
33. Gregory Vlastos, "Justice and Equality," in *Social Justice*, ed. Richard Brandt (Englewood Cliffs: Prentice-Hall, 1962), pp. 31–72.
34. Ibid., p. 53.
35. Ibid., p. 51.
36. Ibid., p. 60.
37. Ibid., p. 54.
38. Richard B. Brandt, *Ethical Theory: The Problems of Normative and Critical Ethics* (Englewood Cliffs: Prentice-Hall, 1959), pp. 434–436.
39. For example, Sissela Bok uses the case of the potential rescuer standing on the wharf to make the point that the rescuer is *not* morally obligated to risk his/her life to save a drowning person unless the rescuer had incurred such an obligation through his/her own prior actions. Sissela Bok, "Ethical Problems of Abortion," *Hastings Center Studies* II (January 1974): 33–52.
40. Polemarchus attributes this saying to the poet Simonides. Plato, *The Republic*, Book I, para. 331. This version of the quote is from the translation by Allan Bloom (New York: Basic Books, 1968), p. 7.
41. Vlastos, "Justice and Equality," p. 55.
42. "Teddy's Tiny World," *Time*, 19 April 1976, pp. 88, 89.
43. Edmond Cahn, *The Sense of Injustice* (Bloomington: Indiana University Press, 1949), especially pp. 11–26.
44. For a discussion of the relationship of duty to the degree of hardship for the actor see Rawls, *Theory of Justice*, pp. 114–117.
45. Frankena disagrees with Vlastos on this point. In Frankena's view, a separate principle of beneficence must be stated. William Frankena, "The Concept of Social Justice," in *Social Justice*, ed. Richard Brandt (Englewood Cliffs: Prentice-Hall, 1962), especially p. 6. In an age of diminishing resources, one may also wonder about the wisdom of advocating consumption at the highest possible level.
46. G. E. M. Anscombe, "Who Is Wronged?" *Oxford Review* V (1967): 16, 17. This case was invented by Philippa Foot, "The Problem of Abortion and the Doctrine of the Double Effect," *Oxford Review* V (1967): 5–15.
47. It may be asked whether this case meets the criteria for our use of the expression *dire* scarcity, because the drug can be further divided and remain effective. But the point here is that for the first patient the drug *cannot* be further divided. In this sense, the scarcity is dire.

48. Anscombe, "Who Is Wronged?" p. 16.
49. Ibid., p. 17.
50. Young also understands Anscombe in this way. He says that Anscombe's remarks "strongly suggest that she would be in sympathy with a 'first-come-first-served' basis." Robert Young, "Some Criteria for Making Decisions Concerning the Distribution of Scarce Medical Resources," *Theory and Decision* VI (1975): 454.

IV. Principles for Triage: The Utilitarian Alternatives

1. It is sometimes thought that impartiality points in the direction of certain substantive principles of practice. Outka, for example, argues that the notion of impartiality "moves us, despite its formality, towards practice." But scrutiny of his argument on this point reveals that Outka is able to make this move because of his already established choice of a *needs* conception of the just distribution of health care. Thus, Outka believes that health care should be distributed equally to those who have equal needs. If it is impossible to provide for the needs of all because, for example, society finds the cost of some treatment too high, then Outka says that persons within a particular disease category should receive impartial treatment. But neither his primary criterion of needs nor his secondary criterion of categories of illness is an entailment of the principle of treating equals equally. Gene Outka, "Social Justice and Equal Access to Health Care," in *Love and Society*, ed. James Johnson and David Smith (Missoula: Scholars Press, 1974), pp. 187–207.
2. See, for example, Ch. Perelman, *The Idea of Justice and the Problem of Argument* (London: Routledge and Kegan Paul, 1963).
3. For a brief discussion of the relation of formal to substantive principles of justice see William Frankena, "The Concept of Social Justice," in *Social Justice*, ed. Richard Brandt (Englewood Cliffs: Prentice-Hall, 1962), pp. 8–9.
4. John Stuart Mill, *Utilitarianism* (New York: Bobbs-Merrill, 1971), p. 44. Sidgwick is another utilitarian whose statement of the principle of impartiality is well known. See Henry Sidgwick, *The Methods of Ethics*, 7th ed. (New York: Dover, 1966), pp. 379–390.
5. Nicholas Rescher, *Distributive Justice: A Constructive Critique of the Utilitarian Theory of Distribution* (New York: Bobbs-Merrill, 1966), p. 73. For similar lists of distributive principles see also John Ryan, *Distributive Justice: The Right and Wrong of Our Present Distribution of Wealth* (New York: Macmillan Company,

1916), chap. 16; John Hospers, *Human Conduct* (New York: Harcourt, Brace and World, 1961) chap. 9; Perelman, *The Idea of Justice*, pp. 17–25.

6. For a strong statement by a physician advocating that the decision making be left to physicians see G. E. Schreiner, "Problems of Ethics in Relation to Haemodialysis and Transplantation," in *Ethics in Medical Progress*, ed. G. E. W. Wolstenholme (Boston: Little, Brown and Company, 1966). See also Frederic B. Westervelt, Jr., "The Selection Process as Viewed from Within: A Reply to Childress," *Soundings* XLVIII (Winter 1970), p. 362.

7. Report of the Fifth Bethesda Conference of the American College of Cardiology, cited in United Nations Economic and Social Council, Commission on Human Rights, "Human Rights and Scientific and Technological Developments," Part II, "Developments in Medicine" (Geneva: June 1975), p. 70 (mimeographed) (hereinafter cited as United Nations, "Human Rights and Scientific Developments.").

8. Leon Kass, "The New Biology: What Price Relieving Man's Estate?" *Science* CLXXIV (19 November 1971), p. 782.

9. A. H. Katz and D. M. Procter, *Social-psychological Characteristics of Patients Receiving Hemodialysis: Treatment for Chronic Renal Failure*, mimeographed (Washington, D.C.: Department of Health, Education, and Welfare, July 1969), p. 23; and Renee C. Fox and Judith P. Swazey, *The Courage to Fail* (Chicago: University of Chicago Press, 1974), p. 243. Obviously such criteria as intelligence tests may also serve indirectly as measures of general social worth. But this was not generally the *expressed* purpose for their use. Rather, they were considered indicators of a candidate's ability to comprehend and follow the treatment regimen.

10. Left aside for the present is the question of whether the elderly were excluded not because the treatment had a low probability of being life-saving but because the number of years of life saved was deemed insufficient.

11. The authors of one article claim, on the basis of their survey of triage practices, that "it is an almost universally accepted standard for selection that the patient whose chances of survival will be most greatly increased by the use of a resource will be preferred over the others." "Scarce Medical Resources," *Columbia Law Review* LXIX (April 1969): 655.

12. Nicholas Rescher, "The Allocation of Exotic Medical Lifesaving Therapy," *Ethics* LXXIX (April 1969): 177.

13. Robert Young, "Some Criteria for Making Decisions Concerning the Distribution of Scarce Medical Resources," *Theory and Decision* VI (1975): 443.

14. David Sanders and Jesse Dukeminier, Jr., "Medical Advance and Legal Lag: Hemodialysis and Kidney Transplantation," *U.C.L.A. Law Review* XV (February, 1968): 379.

15. Ramsey, *The Patient as Person* (New Haven: Yale University Press, 1970), p. 249.

16. Fox and Swazey, *Courage to Fail*, p. 242.
17. Rescher, "Allocation of Lifesaving Therapy," p. 177.
18. Fox and Swazey, *Courage to Fail*, p. 232.
19. Charles Fried, "Rights and Health Care—Beyond Equity and Efficiency," *New England Journal of Medicine* CCXCIII (31 July 1975): 241–245.
20. Fried also calls this a "triage model." In so doing, he is using triage in the limited sense of the efficiency strategy developed in military and disaster medicine.
21. Fried, "Rights and Health Care," p. 243.
22. Ibid., p. 244.
23. Thomas O'Donnell, "The Morality of Triage," *Georgetown Medical Bulletin* XIV (August 1960).
24. In traditional moral theology, questons of priorities under the circumstances of dire scarcity came in the section known as "The Order of Charity." For an example see Henry Davis, S.J., *Human Acts, Law, and Sin*, Vol. I of *Moral and Pastoral Theology*, 2 vols. (New York: Sheed and Ward, 1946), pp. 319 ff. There it is said that a well-ordered charity requires a gradation of the excellence of goods. For example, spiritual needs come before physical needs in most cases, and one should be willing to sacrifice one's own physical life for the spiritual life of another. Needs are graded in three categories: (1) "extreme" need when one is in danger of losing life and cannot help himself or herself, (2) "grave" need when one is in danger and can help himself or herself only with great difficulty, and (3) "common" need when one is able to help himself or herself without much difficulty.
25. O'Donnell, "The Morality of Triage," p. 70.
26. Ibid.
27. See above, chap. 1.
28. Philippa Foot, "The Problem of Abortion and the Doctrine of the the Double Effect," *Oxford Review* V (1967): 9. It should be said that the first concern of Foot's essay is not the allocation of scarce resources but rather the concept of the double effect. Foot chooses not to call her position utilitarian. But her prescription for this case is, nevertheless, in harmony with the utilitarian principle which may be interpreted in this example to mean the greatest good in terms of lives saved for the greatest number of candidates. For a discussion of Anscombe's criticism of Foot's position on allocation, see above, chap. 3.
29. Young, "The Distribution of Scarce Medical Resources," p. 448.
30. For the information on abandonment, I have relied on Neil L. Chayet, *Legal Implications of Emergency Care* (New York: Appleton-Century-Crofts, 1969), especially chap. V, "The Hazards of Abandonment." Chayet says that the charge of abandonment has five elements: "(1) a physician-patient relationship; (2) termination of that relationship by the physician without the mutual consent of the parties; (3) termination without affording the patient the opportunity to secure the ser-

vices of another physician; (4) the patient's continuing need for further treatment by the physician; (5) causal connection between the abandonment and injury or death," p. 194.

31. Ibid., p. 136.
32. Fried, "Rights and Health Care," p. 244.
33. Rescher, "Allocation of Lifesaving Therapy," p. 178.
34. Young, "The Distribution of Scarce Medical Resources," p. 448.
35. Shana Alexander, "They Decide Who Lives, Who Dies: Medical Miracle Puts a Moral Burden on a Small Committee," *Life*, 9 November 1962, p. 123.
36. Robert Nozick, for example, argues that families are "disturbing" for any "patterned" distributive principles of the sort discussed in the present chapter. *Anarchy, State, and Utopia* (New York: Basic Books, 1974), pp. 167–168. And Rawls chooses, for the most part, to conceive of his rational contractors in the "original position" as being heads of families. *Theory of Justice*, pp. 128–129. Rawls makes this move, however, primarily to solve the problems of distribution among various generations and not to derive principles of distribution within a particular generation.
37. For example, Fried takes up a similar problem tangentially in his discussion of the value of life. Charles Fried, *An Anatomy of Values: Problems of Personal and Social Choice* (Cambridge, Mass.: Harvard University Press, 1970), p. 227. He writes: "[S]urely it would be absurd to insist that if a man could, at no risk or cost to himself, save one of two persons in equal peril, and one of those in peril was, say, his wife, he must treat both equally, perhaps by flipping a coin. One answer is that where the potential rescuer occupies no office such as that of captain of a ship, public health official, or the like, the occurrence of the accident may itself stand as a sufficient randomizing event to meet the dictates of fairness, so he may prefer his friend or loved one. Where the rescuer does occupy an official position, the argument that he must overlook personal ties is not unacceptable." What are the just limits of personal bonds such as those of family relationships? Fried says: "One feels that up to a point the personal tie may still be respected, but only up to a point. This issue and the principles it involves remain unresolved for this discussion." Fried's question is obviously different from ours at this point. He is wondering how the decision maker's *own* family ties may legitimately affect his or her moral decisions. He is not concerned in this passage with how the family ties of other people may affect the decision maker. Nevertheless, Fried's discussion, including its inconclusiveness, is illustrative of the difficulty of relating family relationships to the questions of justice.
38. See for example "The Draft: Oh Dad, Poor Dad," *Newsweek* 4 May 1970, p. 28.
39. Ibid. Melvin Laird, then Secretary of Defense, was quoted as saying that an extreme hardship would be "a 19-year-old with five

kids.'' In reality the determination of extreme hardship was left to the local draft boards.

40. The comparison, however, is not original to the present discussion. See Sanders and Dukeminier, ''Medical Advance,'' p. 380. ''A somewhat analogous problem [to that of patient selection], with less drastic consequences from the selection, arises respecting the draft of men to fight wars.''

41. Advocacy of the principle of random selection for triage, or a lottery, is discussed below.

42. Young, ''Scarce Medical Resources,'' p. 654.

43. Rescher, ''Allocation of Lifesaving Therapy,'' p. 178. For a more recent, thoroughgoing defense of using general social worth criteria in triage decision making, see Marc D. Basson, ''Choosing among Candidates for Scarce Medical Resources,'' *Journal of Medicine and Philosophy* 4 (September 1979): 313-333. Basson's basic rationale is identical to Rescher's. Basson writes: '' 'Society' is just a large group of people and, like any group of people, may dispose of its resources as it sees fit, for the maximal benefit of its members,'' p. 318.

44. Rescher, ''Allocation of Lifesaving Therapy,'' p. 178.

45. James Childress, ''Who Shall Live When Not All Can Live?'' *Soundings* XLIII (Winter, 1970), pp. 339-362. For a theological argument against the possibility of human beings making accurate appraisals of other human beings' social worth, see Helmut Thielicke, ''The Doctor as Judge of Who Shall Live and Who Shall Die,'' *Who Shall Live*, ed. Kenneth Vaux (Philadelphia: Fortress Press, 1970), especially pp. 171-174. Thielicke makes a case for the human being's ''alien dignity.'' ''The basis of human dignity is seen to reside not in any immanent quality of man whatsoever, but in the fact that God created him. Man is the apple of God's eye,'' p. 172. Thielicke argues against seeking *any* objective criteria for triage decision making. ''Whoever seeks for such criteria, by that very fact—though perhaps without his even knowing it—has already surrendered to the utilitarian point of view. He has attempted to apply quantitative standards to that which, because it bears the quality of the unconditional, simply cannot be measured. And in so doing he has missed the very point of the humanum, the alien dignity,'' p. 172.

46. Childress, ''Who Shall Live?'' p. 346.

47. Joseph Fletcher, ''Donor Nephrectomies and Moral Responsibility,'' *Journal of the American Medical Women's Association* XXIII (December 1968): 1085-1091. A similar argument for developing more accurate measurements of social worth for the purpose of triage is offered by Basson, ''Choosing Among Candidates.''

48. Fletcher, ''Donor Nephrectomies,'' p. 1090.

49. Childress, ''Who Shall Live?'' pp. 348-349.

50. Ramsey, *Patient as Person*, p. 255. Ramsey's line of argument is similar in many ways to both Childress, ''Who Shall Live?'' and

Thielicke, "Who Shall Live and Who Shall Die." Childress also calls for a random approach to selection, and he also equated the lottery with the queue. Thielicke is often interpreted as calling for a random approach, but his prescription is less clear. He does say: "Since these [various objective] criteria are, as we have indicated, questionable, necessarily alien to the meaning of human existence, the decision to which they lead can be little more than that arrived at by casting lots." (p. 174). But then he goes on to suggest that various objective criteria must be taken into account. He says, for example, that "there are economic factors to be considered, involving the patient as well as other public or private sources of funds. These and many other considerations could be decisive" (p. 174). His main point seems to be that we should "keep open the wound, to preserve the ambiguity, and so to remain faithful to an awareness of that which is human" (p. 174). Perhaps the practical aspects of his argument are best understood as an attempt to preserve ambiguity.

51. Rescher, "Allocation of Lifesaving Therapy," p. 178.

52. Ibid., p. 179. Basson argues that "all" of Rescher's selection criteria are "merely facets of the broader notion of social utility." "Choosing Among Candidates," p. 330. But this assertion is incorrect. It is, of course, possible to argue for rewarding past performance on the grounds that such rewards maximize social utility. But it is also possible to do as Rescher does and argue for just rewards on the basis of a principle of equity.

53. Ibid., p. 185.

54. Leo Shatin, a professor of psychiatry whose advocacy of the principle of general social worth was discussed briefly in chapter 1, is one of the "others." It will be remembered that Shatin, in his essay, "Medical Care and the Social Worth of Man," claimed that evaluations of social worth are inevitable so we should be honest about such evaluations and try to make them as rational as possible.

55. In a report submitted to the United Nations Commission on Human Rights, the Government of Romania made the following statement: "The Government of Romania considers that beneficiaries of advanced medical techniques should be first of all young people and persons of high esteem or endowed with certain creative possibilities such as famous inventors, scientists and statesmen." United Nations Economic and Social Council, Commission on Human Rights, "Human Rights and Scientific and Technological Developments," Part II, "Developments in Medicine," mimeographed (Geneva: June 1975), p. 75.

V.   Principles for Triage: The Egalitarian Alternatives

1. David Miller, *Social Justice* (Oxford: Clarendon Press, 1976), p. 149.
2. Paul Ramsey, *Patient as Person* (New Haven: Yale University Press, 1970), p. 260.
3. G. E. M. Anscombe, "Who Is Wronged?" *Oxford Review* V (1967): 16.
4. For example see the discussion of the Talmudic literature in Immanuael Jakobvits, *Jewish Medical Ethics* (New York: Bloch Publishing Company, 1959), pp. 97–98. "The deliberate sacrifice of a human life is unlawful even if it may save many other people from certain death," p. 98.
5. Philosophical interest in such cases does not seem to have waned. See, for example, Alan Donagan's discussion of cases of necessity in *The Theory of Morality* (Chicago: University of Chicago Press, 1977), pp. 172–180. Donagan argues that common morality forbids saving some lives at the expense of other lives. Thus, one cannot save one's own life if it means taking the life of an innocent (that it, nonaggressive) other. But Donagan makes an exception in the oft-discussed case of the "trapped potholers." Donagan says that common morality would permit the trapped potholers to blow up one of their comrades in order to free themselves. This is so, he argues, because there is at least a tacit agreement among people who undertake such hazardous pastimes that should such an emergency arise it would be permissible to save the largest possible number of lives. But Donagan goes on to say that it would not be morally acceptable to free a trapped group if it meant blowing up an innocent and unsuspecting group of picnickers. For a criticism of this argument see Bernard Gert, review of *The Theory of Morality* by Alan Donagan, in *Journal of Medicine and Philosophy* II (December 1977): 410–419.
6. Edmond Cahn, *The Moral Decision: Right and Wrong in the Light of American Law* (Bloomington: Indiana University Press, 1955), pp. 61–71. The official citation for this case is *United States v. Holmes*, 26 Fed. Cas. 360 (C.C.E.D. Pa. 1842). Both Childress and Ramsey also consider Cahn's discussion of *Holmes*. See James Childress, "Who Shall Live When Not All Can Live?" *Soundings* XLIII (Winter 1970): 341–343 and Ramsey, *Patient as Person*, pp. 259–266.
7. *Holmes*, 26 Fed. Cas. 367.
8. Cahn, *The Moral Decision*, p. 71. Cahn does not cite the reference, but it seems he is reflecting a passage from *Mishnah Sanhedrin* 4:5: "For this reason was one single man created: to teach you that anyone who destroys a single life is as though he destroyed the whole of mankind; and anyone who preserves a

single life is as though he preserved the whole of mankind." For a compilation of Jewish rabbinical statements that may have relevance for the type of case represented by *Holmes*, see Sid Z. Leiman, "The Sinking of the *William Brown*: A Case Study in Jewish Ethics," unpublished paper, 1975).

9. Cahn, *The Moral Decision*, p. 71.

10. *Queen* v. *Dudley and Stephens*, 14 Q. B. D. 273 (1884). This case is also discussed by Cahn in another work: Edmond Cahn, *The Sense of Injustice* (Bloomington: Indiana University Press, 1949), p. 29. And the case is taken up by Donagan in his discussion of necessity. *Theory of Morality*, pp. 175–177.

11. Dudley and Stephens were sentenced to death, but according to the official record: "This sentence was afterwards commuted by the Crown to six months' imprisonment." *Dudley*, 14 Q. B. D. 288.

12. In the judge's words: "[W]hile we admit that sailor and sailor may lawfully struggle with each other for the plank which can save but one, we think that, if the passenger is on the plank, even the 'law of necessity' justifies not the sailor who takes it from him." *Holmes*, 26 Fed. Cas. 367.

13. Information furnished by the Government of Austria, November 21, 1974, quoted in United Nations Economic and Social Council, Commission on Human Rights, "Human Rights and Scientific and Technological Developments," Part II, "Developments in Medicine," mimeographed (Geneva: June 1975), p. 74.

14. Left aside at this point is the question of whether it may ever be economically feasible to provide some types of medical care to all who are in need.

15. *The Totally Implantable Artificial Heart: Economic, Ethical, Legal, Medical, Psychiatric, Social Implications* (Washington, D.C.: Department of Health, Education, and Welfare, 1973), p. 142, hereinafter called *Artificial Heart*.

16. Miller, *Social Justice*, p. 149.

17. Robert M. Veatch, "What is 'Just' Health Care Delivery?" in *Ethics and Health Policy*, ed. Robert M. Veatch and Roy Branson (Cambridge, Mass.: Ballinger Publishing Company, 1976), p. 142.

18. Ibid., p. 133.

19. Ibid., p. 141.

20. Bernard Williams, "The Idea of Equality," in *Justice and Equality*, ed. Hugo Bedau (Englewood Cliffs: Prentice-Hall, 1971), p. 127.

21. Veatch briefly discusses disaster triage in "What is 'Just' Health Care Delivery?" p. 136. There he defends what we have called the principle of immediate usefulness (U-2).

22. Edward P. Joyce, private interview, 2 August 1976.

23. Veatch, "What is 'Just' Health Care Delivery?" p. 134.

24. It would seem that Veatch's argument would be considerably clearer on this point if he distinguished between the "sickest " and the medically "neediest." Veatch does not bother to define

"sickest." Does it mean those patients suffering the greatest amount of pain? Those with the severest disabilities? Or those nearest death? But whatever the definition, it is clear that it cannot be automatically inferred that the sickest *need* the available medical resources. At least some of the sickest are likely to be beyond the point where medical care can prevent further harm, except perhaps some of the harm of pain and suffering. What point is there, then, in raising (as Veatch does) the specter of the incurably ill exhausting *all* of the medical resources? Unless Veatch is talking about medical research, and he does not seem to be, the incurably ill, by definition, do not *need* most of the medical resources presently available. But enough has already been said on earlier pages about the relationship of the concept of needs to the probability of avoiding harm. What is lacking in Veatch's discussion is not only a definition of "sickest" but also some analysis of what it means to be the "neediest."

25. Hans Jonas, "Philosophical Reflections on Experimenting with Human Subjects," in *Experimentation with Human Subjects*, ed. Paul A. Freund (New York: George Braziller, 1969), p. 23.
26. This was at least partially the case with the Seattle center. In order to be included in the center's home dialysis program, the patients had to demonstrate an ability to pay $11,000 initially and $250 per month for three years. "Scarce Medical Resources," *Columbia Law Review* LXIX (April 1969): 652. But even in the Seattle center, financial need sometimes had the opposite effect. Murray reported the selection of one working-class candidate whose large family had serious financial needs. J. Murray et al., "A Community Hemodialysis Center for the Treatment of Chronic Uremia," *Transactions: American Society for Artificial Internal Organs* VII (1962): 316. From the information given, however, it is difficult to tell whether the main concern was the candidate's financial need or the potential burden on society if the candidate's family had become dependent on public support.
27. Information supplied by Nancy Raby and cited in "Scarce Medical Resources," p. 652. A similar policy was followed at one Los Angeles center.
28. Gregory Vlastos, "Justice and Equality," in *Social Justice*, ed. Richard Brandt (Englewood Cliffs: Prentice-Hall, 1962), p. 51.
29. Veatch makes this point in his comparison of the good of health care with the good of liberty: "One cannot trade off liberty for other goods, because liberty by its very nature is required for enjoyment of the others. Health is, in some ways, like liberty. Certainly death-preventing medical care is like liberty in this respect." Veatch, "What is 'Just' Health Care Delivery?", p. 137.
30. Robert M. Veatch, "Models for Ethical Medicine in a Revolutionary Age," *Hastings Center Report* II (June 1972): 7.
31. This point is made in "Patient Selection for Artificial and Transplanted Organs," *Harvard Law Review* LXXXII (1969): 1342 (hereinafter cited as "Patient Selection").

32. There are exceptions, of course. For example, it is sometimes deemed necessary to move a patient from an intensive care unit in order to make room for another patient with greater needs who arrives later.

33. Charles Fried, *Medical Experimentation: Personal Integrity and Social Policy* (New York: American Elsevier Publishing Company, 1974), pp. 132–137. It should also be noted that Childress argues that random selection, which he equates with queuing, is a method that best preserves relationships of trust. "Who Shall Live?" p. 349.

34. Ibid., p. 137.

35. For a list of institutions that followed the practice of first come, first served see "Scarce Medical Resources," pp. 659–660. The list includes some of the larger medical centers such as Georgetown University Hospital and Yale-New Haven Hospital.

36. Emil Brunner, *Justice and the Social Order*, trans. Mary Hottinger (New York: Harper and Brothers, 1945), p. 29.

37. Ramsey, *Patient as Person*, p. 252; Childress, "Who Shall Live?" p. 353.

38. Ramsey, *Patient as Person*, p. 252.

39. Ramsey, for example, says: "[R]andom patient selection can be instituted, either by lottery or by a policy of 'first come, first served.' " *Patient as Person*, p. 252. And Childress says: "My proposal is that we use some form of randomness or chance (either natural, such as 'first come, first served,' or artificial, such as a lottery) to determine who shall be saved." "Who Shall Live?" p. 347. Other examples of the equation of randomness with queuing are found in the following: "Artificial Heart," p. 148; "Scarce Medical Resources," pp. 659–660; Young, "Some Criteria for Making Decisions Concerning the Distribution of Scarce Medical Resources," *Theory and Decision* VI (1975): 445. In the following chapter it will be argued that this equation is erroneous.

40. This objection is raised by Gerald Leach in *The Biocrats: Ethics and the New Medicine* (Baltimore: Penguin Books, 1972), p. 259.

41. "Artificial Heart," p. 148.

42. "Scarce Medical Resources," p. 660.

43. Ibid.

44. Ibid. The same report says, for example, that random selection at one New York facility led to the treatment of "a narcotics addict and a homosexual" much to the stress of one of the physicians who saw "deserving patients" rejected while others were saved for "an unhappy or anti-social life."

45. Childress, "Who Shall Live?" p. 348.

46. Paul Freund, "Introduction," in *Experimentation with Human Subjects*, ed. Paul Freund (New York: George Braziller, 1970), p. xvii.

47. For an extended discussion of the ethics of randomized clinical trials see Fried, *Medical Experimentation*.

48. Robert Platt, "Ethical Problems in Medical Procedures," in

Ethics in Medical Progress: With Special Reference to Transplantation (Boston: Little, Brown and Company, 1966), pp. 150–151. Platt recognizes the potential moral problem of combining the functions of research and therapy. "There is a slight ethical danger here, in that one is selecting patients for such procedures partly because they may benefit other people in the future and not wholly because of possible benefit to the present patient," p. 151.

49. For a careful discussion of the necessary distinctions among these three concepts see Karen Lebacqz, "Reflections on the Report and Recommendations of the National Commission: Research on the Fetus," *Villanova Law Review* XXII (1976–1977): 357–383.

50. Shana Alexander, "They Decide Who Lives, Who Dies: Medical Miracle Puts a Moral Burden on a Small Committee," *Life* 9 November 1962, p. 123. One senses a similar, albeit veiled, criticism in a comment by Fox and Swazey: "[O]ne can raise the question whether the use of methods such as first-come, first-served and random selection represent an abdication of the decision-making responsibilities that are an inherent part of the physician's role." Renee C. Fox and Judith P. Swazey, *The Courage to Fail* (Chicago: University of Chicago Press, 1974), p. 270. For another statement of this and other criticisms of random selection, see Marc D. Basson, "Choosing Among Candidates for Scarce Medical Resources," *Journal of Medicine and Philosophy* 4 (September 1979): 313–333.

51. Leach, *The Biocrats*, p. 260.

52. Leo Shatin, "Medical Care and the Social Worth of Man," *American Journal of Orthopsychiatry* XXXVI (1966): 100.

53. Charles Fried, "Equality and Rights in Medical Care," *Hastings Center Report* VI (February 1976): 29–37. Fried argues that everyone in society should be provided with what he calls a "decent minimum" of health care. Beyond this, people should be free to purchase whatever health care they choose. On this view, society definitely does not have an obligation to provide the best possible health care for the entire citizenry. To attempt to do so, Fried argues, would inevitably lower the quality of health care available to some and also "carry us over a reasonable budget limit," ibid., p. 30. Since TIAH would be one of the health care items Fried would not include in a "decent minimum" but would not want to prohibit, it seems clear that Fried's method of allocation would be based on the candidate's ability to pay. Obviously, this method of distribution also suffers from boundary problems. Would candidates, say, from some of the oil-rich nations be able to buy the entire supply even though the citizens of another country paid taxes that helped develop the devices?

54. Ibid., p. 31.

55. Young, "The Distribution of Scarce Medical Resources," p. 452.

56. The language of "methodological presumption" and "burden of proof" is borrowed primarily from J. Philip Wogaman. See generally his *A Christian Method of Moral Judgment*

(Philadelphia: Westminster Press, 1976). Such expressions, however, are also commonly used by other ethicists and philosophers of law. See, for example, Rawls, *Theory of Justice* (Cambridge: Harvard University Press, 1971), p. 507.

57. Young, "The Distribution of Scarce Medical Resources," p. 452. A somewhat similar stance is taken by Rescher. He introduces random selection only after a long list of other criteria, mostly utilitarian in nature, have been considered. Nicholas Rescher, "The Allocation of Exotic Medical Lifesaving Therapy," *Ethics* LXXIX (April 1969).

58. Ramsey, *Patient as Person*, p. 239.

59. Ibid., p. 249.

60. James Childress, "Rationing of Medical Treatment," in *The Encyclopedia of Bioethics*, vol. 4, ed. Warren T. Reich (New York: Free Press, 1978), p. 1417.

VI. Justice as Fairness

1. For a remarkably clear example see William Frankena, *Ethics*, 2d ed. (Englewood Cliffs: Prentice-Hall, 1973), pp. 34–52.

2. Of the examples of this approach that come to mind, perhaps the clearest statement is Nicholas Rescher's *Distributive Justice: A Constructive Critique of the Utilitarian Theory of Distribution* (New York: Bobbs-Merrill Company, 1966). Other examples include: Richard B. Brandt, *Ethical Theory: The Problems of Normative and Critical Ethics* (Englewood Cliffs: Prentice-Hall, 1959), see especially Chap. XVI, pp. 407–32; and Norman E. Bowie, *Towards a New Theory of Distributive Justice* (Amherst: University of Massachusetts Press, 1971), see especially Chap. V. Bowie would probably object to being listed among those who advocate an *intuitive* balancing of equality and utility. He attempts to work out an elaborate system that would make distributive justice a weighing of numerous factors including liberty, equality, hapiness, efficiency, and merit. On this view, the relative weight of each factor would depend on circumstances such as the society's relative level of affluence. But, in spite of Bowie's operose discussion of the problems of priority, the ordinal rank of each factor remains very largely intuitive.

3. Rawls, *Theory of Justice* (Cambridge: Harvard University Press, 1971), p. 40.

4. One exception, it would appear, is R. M. Hare. See his "Rawls' Theory of Justice," *Philosophical Quarterly* XXIII (April and July 1973): 144 ff. and 241 ff. Reprinted in *Reading Rawls: Critical Studies on Rawls' 'A Theory of Justice,'* ed. Norman Daniels (New York: Basic Books, 1974), pp. 81–107. Additional references

to Hare's essay are from this reprinted version. Hare may not go so far as to call Rawls's work unimportant, but Hare argues that Rawls's theory is very much like "ideal observer" theories. Thus, according to Hare, Rawls adds nothing particularly new to our moral understanding.

5. Brian Barry, *The Liberal Theory of Justice* (Oxford: Clarendon Press, 1973), p. ix.

6. See, for example, Roger D. Masters, "Is Contract an Adequate Basis for Medical Ethics?" *Hastings Center Report* V (December 1975): 24–28. It should be noted that Masters is working with a somewhat broader notion of contract than is Rawls. In fact, Masters never cites Rawls, which seems somewhat odd in light of his references to other contract theorists from Glaucon to Locke and even Paul Ramsey. An important essay which questions the possibility of using Rawls's work to develop a theory of justice for health care is Norman Daniels, "Rights to Health Care and Distributive Justice: Programmatic Worries," *Journal of Medicine and Philosophy* 4 (1979): 174–191.

7. A notable exception which has informed the present work is Ronald M. Green, "Health Care and Justice in Contract Theory Perspective," in *Ethics and Health Policy*, ed. Robert M. Veatch and Roy Branson (Cambridge, Mass.: Ballinger Publishing Company, 1976), pp. 111–126. It should also be noted that Childress depends on a Rawlsian perspective at certain key points in his discussion of scarce medical resources. See James Childress, "Who Shall Live When Not All Can Live?" *Soundings* XLIII (Winter 1970), pp. 350 ff. Other discussions of justice and health care delivery occasionally mention Rawls's theory in brief sections. See, for example, Robert M. Veatch, "What is 'Just' Health Care Delivery?" in *Ethics and Health Policy*, ed. Robert M. Veatch and Roy Branson (Cambridge, Mass.: Ballinger Publishing Company, 1976), pp. 134–136, and Alastair V. Campbell, *Medicine, Health and Justice: The Problem of Priorities* (Edinburgh: Churchill Livingstone, 1978), pp. 73–84.

8. Nozick, *Anarchy, State, and Utopia* (New York: Basic Books, 1974), p. 183.

9. Rawls, *Theory of Justice*, especially Chap. III.

10. Ibid., pp. 136–142.

11. Ibid., pp. 90–95.

12. Perhaps the best known contemporary statement of this type of theory is Roderick Firth, "Ethical Absolutism and the Ideal Observer," *Philosophy and Phenomenological Research* XII (1952): 317–345.

13. "Whatever you wish that men would do to you, do so to them; for this is the law and the prophets." Matthew 7:12 (Revised Standard Version).

14. For Rawls's discussion of the advantages of the weaker stipulations see *Theory of Justice*, pp. 148–149. Rawls takes special

pains to distinguish the mutual disinterestedness of the original position from various egoistic theories, pp. 124, 135 ff., and 147 ff. He says, for example: "The motivation of the persons in the original position must not be confused with the motivation of persons in everyday life who accept the principles that would be chosen and who have the corresponding sense of justice. In practical affairs an individual does have a knowledge of his situation and he can, if he wishes, exploit contingencies to his advantage. Should his sense of justice move him to act on the principles of right that would be adopted in the original position, his desires and aims are surely not egoistic. He voluntarily takes on the limitations expressed by this interpretation of the moral point of view," p. 148.

15. Probably the best known text on game theory is R. Duncan Luce and Howard Raiffa, *Games and Decisions: Introduction and Critical Survey* (New York: Wiley, 1957). For a discussion of Rawls's theory in the light of game theory, see Robert Paul Wolff, *Understanding Rawls: A Reconstruction and Critique of 'A Theory of Justice'* (Princeton: Princeton University Press, 1977), pp. 50–56.

16. Rawls, *Theory of Justice*, pp. 14–15; see also pp. 60–64.

17. Ibid., p. 302. "Lexical" is Rawls's word for the notion of a rank ordering of the principles such that the principle given first priority must be fully applied before moving to the application of the principle of second priority, and so on through the list of principles. In the simplified list given here, IIa and IIb are reversed from the order given by Rawls. This is done because Rawls gives priority to the principle of equal opportunity over the difference principle. It also should be noted that this simplified version does not include Rawls's "just savings principle," which governs the distribution of resources among generations.

18. Ibid., pp. 8–9, and p. 245–246.

19. Ibid., pp. 126–130. Rawls follows Hume in the matter of moderate scarcity. For a discussion of Hume's position, see chap. 3 above.

20. Ibid., pp. 243–251, and pp. 541–548.

22. Ibid., p. 543.

23. Rawls's arguments for the ranking of equality of opportunity are difficult to extract. Indeed, in commenting on this difficulty, one critic remarks: "[T]he reader who sets himself to comprehend the precise relation between the elements in Rawls's theory should not be surprised if he notices steam coming out of his ears." Brian Barry, *The Liberal Theory of Justice* (Oxford: Clarendon Press, 1973), p. 84. The analysis in the present discussion is based primarily on what are taken to be Rawls's main treatments of the issue. Rawls, *Theory of Justice*, pp. 83–90, 298–301, and 511–512.

23. Rawls, *Theory of Justice*, p. 84.

24. For a discussion of the possible interpretations and a critique of Rawls's position see Wolff, *Understanding Rawls*, pp. 41, 47–49.
25. Rawls, *Theory of Justice*, p. 73.
26. Ibid., p. 15.
27. Ibid., pp. 100–101.
28. Ibid., p. 153.
29. Ibid., p. 154.
30. Ibid., p. 303.
31. Ibid., p. 279.
32. Ibid., p. 126–129.
33. Ibid., p. 127. [Emphasis added.]
34. Ibid., p. 7.
35. Ibid., p. 55.
36. Albert R. Jonsen and Andre E. Hellegers, "Conceptual Foundations for an Ethics of Medical Care," in *Ethics of Health Care*, ed. Laurence R. Tancredi (Washington, D.C.: National Academy of Sciences, 1974), p. 14. The authors define an institution as 'a complex interaction of professionals, paraprofessionals, and the public, on informational, economic, and occupational levels, in identifiable physical environments, whose coordinated decisions and actions have magnified public impact and is recognized culturally and legally as affecting the public welfare in a significant way," p. 14.
37. Rawls, *Theory of Justice*, p. 8. Rawls rejects what he calls an "allocative conception of justice" in which goods are allotted on the basis of some scheme that ignores established expectations. With this view, Rawls claims, "Justice becomes a kind of efficiency, unless equality is preferred," p. 88. In contrast, the pure procedural justice of contract theory calls for a distribution of goods based on legitimate expectations which have grown out of institutions of social cooperation. See also p. 64.
38. Wolff, *Understanding Rawls*, p. 77.
39. Nozick, *Anarchy, State and Utopia*, p. 204.
40. Ibid., p. 206.
41. For criticism of Nozick's remarks on this subject see Thomas Nagel, "Libertarianism without Foundations," *Yale Law Review* LXXXV (1975): 139–141.
42. It is interesting to note that Nozick uses the illustration of academic grading in an attempt to refute the decision-making conditions of the original position. *Anarchy, State, and Utopia*, pp. 199–201. The grading example, and Nozick's discussion of it, serve well to demonstrate the inadequacy of using any and every small-scale social practice to test principles for the basic social structure.
43. Rawls, *Theory of Justice*, p. 96: "I suppose, then, that for the most part each person holds two relevant positions: that of equal citizenship and that defined by his place in the distribution of income and wealth." This is a simplification which Rawls argues is

197

necessary in order to have a "coherent and manageable theory," p. 96. It is not hard to understand why Rawls decided to focus the discussion in this manner. There would no doubt be an unmanageable number of complications if an attempt were made to compare the status of the least advantaged person in terms of each major social institution and then concoct a comprehensive index for all representative positions. Nevertheless, Rawls's suggestion that positions other than those of wealth and citizenship are entered voluntarily and, therefore, do not require the same analysis is far from convincing.

44. Ibid., p. 101.
45. Ibid., p. 111.
46. For a discussion of the relationship between such social factors and health see Victor R. Fuchs, *Who Shall Live? Health, Economics, and Social Choice* (New York: Basic Books, 1974), especially Chap. II, "Who Shall Live?" pp. 30–55. Fuchs demonstrated that levels of education and income are more likely to affect some indices of health such as infant mortality than is medical care.
47. In fact, this argument has become quite commonplace in recent times. See, for example, Aaron Wildavsky; "Doing Better and Feeling Worse: The Political Pathology of Health Policy," in *Doing Better and Feeling Worse: Health in the United States*, ed. John H. Knowles (New York: W. W. Norton and Company, 1977), pp. 105–123. See also Fuchs, *Who Shall Live?* pp. 52–55. One of the best known arguments of this sort is Ivan Illich, *Medical Nemesis: The Expropriation of Health* (New York: Pantheon Books, 1976). Unfortunately this work is often long on rhetoric and footnotes and short on accuracy.
48. Green, "Health Care and Justice," p. 112.
49. Ibid.
50. Veatch makes this same point: "[I]t could be argued that health is a prior requirement for receipt of any other goods. Rawls has argued that liberty is such a good. One cannot trade off liberty for other goods, because liberty by its very nature is required for enjoyment of the others. Health is, in some ways, like liberty. Certainly death-preventing medical care is like liberty in this respect." "What is 'Just' Health Care Delivery?" p. 137.
51. Daniels, "Rights to Health Care." See especially pp. 184–186.
52. It also should be noted that Daniels contends that if health care is included in the list of primary social goods, the problem of trade-offs between health care and other goods must be faced. As Daniels observes: "Man does not live by good health care alone, nor is it what makes life worth living. So we can suppose contractors will want to allow for the development and distribution of other goods, even at the expense of reducing investment in health care," ibid., p. 186.
The problem of trade-offs is obviously serious and immensely complicated. To date, I have seen no satisfactory solutions. If the

present goal were to construct a general theory of justice for health care, some attempt at a solution would be essential. But our discussion is limited to principles of microallocation for scarce life-saving resources once socially cooperative efforts have made them available. Even with life-saving health care in the list of social primary goods, Rawlsian contractors might for example, elect to forgo the development of an artificial heart in favor of some other social good. Still, I have no doubt that rational contractors would place a very high priority on the development and provision of death-preventing health care. While it is true that people do not live by good health care alone, without life-saving health care they may not live at all. But, as important as the task may be, I make no attempt in this work to state a principle that should govern the trade-offs essential to macroallocation decisions.

53. Consider, for example, Aristotle's discussion of slaves and women in *The Politics*, Book I, Chap. II–IV.

54. There have been notable exceptions. J. S. Mill, for example insisted that the happiness of "all sentient beings" is morally significant. See for instance his *A System of Logic*, vol. 1: *On the Logic of the Moral Sciences*, chap. 7.

55. See for example Peter Singer, *Animal Liberation: A New Ethics for Our Treatment of Animals* (New York: New York Review, 1974). See also the series of articles in *Ethics* LXXXVIII (January 1978), 95–138.

56. Nozick, *Anarchy, State and Utopia*, p. 39.

57. Rawls, *Theory of Justice*, pp. 17–22, 126–127, 504–512.

58. Ibid., p. 510.

59. Ibid., p. 505. "One should observe that moral personality is here defined as a potentiality that is ordinarily realized in due course. It is this potentiality which brings the claims of justice into play." (For criticism of Rawls on the status of children see Hare, "Rawls's Theory of Justice," pp. 99–100.)

60. Ibid., p. 508.

61. Ibid., pp. 17, 504–505, and 512. This does not mean that there are no moral obligations to animals. But Rawls contends that such obligations are not properly included in a theory of justice.

62. Ibid., p. 506.

63. Ibid. This argument may sound strangely utilitarian for one who has cast his theory in terms of an alternative to utilitarianism. If this particular aspect of the argument is properly called utilitarian, then it must be some sort of rule-utilitarianism of the "Ideal" sort. For a discussion of this classification see David Lyons, *Forms and Limits of Utilitarianism* (Oxford: Clarendon Press, 1965), especially p. 172–173. The difference between teleological and deontological theories seems, at times, to hinge on terminology. Rawls says: "All ethical doctrines worth our attention take consequences into account in judging rightness. One which did not would simply be irrational, crazy." *Theory of*

Justice, p. 30. The main consequence Rawls's theory takes into account is the establishment and preservation of just social institutions. Thus the "good of justice" is given priority over other goods such as happiness or pleasure. The rational contractors in Rawls's theory do not think of just institutions as "maximizing the good." But, of course, if an "ideal rule-utilitarianism" made the good of justice its highest good, it might be difficult to distinguish its basic justification from that of Rawls's theory.

64. This is not to say that there are no societal boundary problems with disaster triage. One of the difficulties encountered in triage planning for disasters, at least in the United States, is that there are multiple levels of policy making institutions including local, state, and federal governmental agencies. Often there are overlapping jurisdictions, and seldom are there definitive guidelines setting forth the relationship of an agency at one level to some other agency at a different level.

65. See, for example, *Transactions: American Society for Artificial Internal Organs* XXII (1976). Even though this journal is the product of an American society, reports are also included of work done on various aspects of the artificial heart in a number of different nations, including Japan, West Germany, and Canada. In some of these cases, the research is supported by the national governments.

66. Shana Alexander, "They Decide Who Lives, Who Dies: Medical Miracle Puts a Moral Burden on a Small Committee," *Life* 9 November 1962, p. 107.

67. For a detailed account of the social and political factors in the development of renal dialysis, including the sources of financial support, see Richard A. Rettig, *Health Care Technology: Lessons Learned from the End-Stage Renal Disease Experience* (Santa Monica: Rand Corporation, 1976).

68. Alexander, "They Decide," p. 108.

69. Rawls, *Theory of Justice*, pp. 8, 126–127.

70. Ibid., pp. 377–378. This is Rawls's only passage on international justice, and it comes in the context of a discussion of conscientious objection to participation in war. (For criticism of Rawls on international relations see Barry, *Liberal Theory of Justice*, pp. 128–133).

71. Ibid., pp. 132–133. For a longer discussion of similar formal criteria see Brandt, *Ethical Theory*, pp. 16–36.

72. For example, it was reported that an organization of Dutch heart patients is sponsoring charter flights to Houston, Texas, where the members undergo open heart surgery for an all-inclusive price of $10,000. "Dutch Seek U. S. Heart Surgery," *Daily Californian* 13 May 1976, p. 2.

73. In the United States, for example, health care institutions may be run by local, state, or federal agencies, or they may be operated by nongovernmental organizations. Some of these institutions are prohibited by law from offering services to persons outside certain

boundaries such as a county or outside certain classifications such as veterans. For a discussion of this problem see "Scarce Medical Resources," *Columbia Law Review* LXIX (April 1969): 640–643.

74. Even in a nation such as Great Britain with its National Health Service, there are gross inequities among the various regions. For example, in the North Western region the percentage of patients who had waited for more than a year to receive needed treatment was significantly higher than the national average. "Waiting Lists Lengthen," *Lancet* I (January 15, 1977): 152.

VII. Triage and Justice

1. Left aside is the problem of making decisions for those who are unable to express their own rational preferences. Lacking definite evidence about the person's choice, contract theory would call for us to decide on the person's behalf as we would decide for ourselves in the original position. For a discussion of this problem see Karen Tait and Gerald Winslow, "Beyond Consent—The Ethics of Decision Making in Emergency Medicine," *Western Journal of Medicine* CXXVI (February 1977): 156–159.

2. This point has been raised by Calabresi. With regard to scarce renal dialysis, he writes: "The lottery treats the man who wants to live desperately, even with an artificial kidney, exactly in the same way as the man who other things being equal might prefer to live but for whom the burden of an artificial kidney (or of life in general) is such that he would almost as soon die." Guido Calabresi, *Memorandum* (1970), p. 20. Cited in Jay Katz and Alexander M. Capron, *Catastrophic Diseases: Who Decides What?* (New York: Russell Sage Foundation, 1975), p. 193.

3. Rawls, *Theory of Justice*, p. 15.

4. Marc D. Basson, "Choosing Among Candidates for Scarce Medical Resources," *Journal of Medicine and Philosophy* 4 (September 1979): 322.

5. Rawls, *Theory of Justice*, p. 128. "Head of family" might not always mean the same as "parent." But the context in which Rawls is using the expression would indicate that the two are synonymous.

6. It might be argued, of course, that contractors who knew they were parents would not choose principles favoring parents *if* they were also trying to protect their children's access to the scarce resources. When the veil is lifted, they might discover that their children were among the ones needing the goods. But this argument does not remove the danger of partiality. The contractors could choose principles favoring parents and children with living parents, since the contractors know that they themselves are living and have children. The effect of such principles would be to rule out nonparents whose own parents were deceased.

201

7. Whether Rawls actually solves this problem would, of course, be sharply contested. See, for example, Robert Paul Wolff, *Understanding Rawls: A Reconstruction and Critique of 'A Theory of Justice'* (Princeton University Press, 1977), pp. 95–98.
8. Rawls, *Theory of Justice*, pp. 167–175.
9. As would be expected, Rawls has been roundly criticized for attributing to the contractors those characteristics which would, in turn, guarantee the selection of principles in harmony with Rawls's own antiutilitarian intuitions. Hare, for example says: "[T]he very most that Rawls may have done towards setting up a non-utilitarian theory of justice is to show that it is possible, if one desires, so to rig the assumptions of the theory that it does not lead straight to a utilitarian conclusion." R. M. Hare, "Rawls' Theory of Justice," *Philosophical Quarterly* XXIII (April and July 1973): 104. Hare and others have found Rawlsian contractors' attitudes toward risk-probability calculations to be unnatural or irrational. See for example, David Lyons, "Nature and Soundness of the Contract and Coherence Arguments," in *Reading Rawls*, ed. Norman Daniels (New York: Basic Books, 1975), pp. 141–167.
10. In fact, probability calculations would appear to be necessary at a number of points in Rawls's theory. For example, Lyons points out that the discovery of which goods are primary would require some sort of probabilistic reasoning. "Contract and Coherence Arguments," p. 162.
11. Left aside are the problems of fiduciary relationships and abandonment. The assumption is made here that the needs of the candidates have become known at roughly the same time and the treatment of none of them has yet begun.
12. Ramsey is correct in suggesting that Cahn's rejection of random selection of survivors appears to be based on the false equation of a lottery with "saving oneself." *Patient as Person* (New Haven: Yale University Press, 1970), p. 262.
13. Ronald M. Green, "Health Care and Justice in Contract Theory Perspective," in *Ethics and Health Policy*, ed. Robert M. Veatch and Roy Branson (Cambridge, Mass.: Ballinger Publishing Company, 1976), p. 117. Left aside is the issue of potential conflicts between basic liberties and health care. Green contends that there is little reason to expect such conflicts. But from the perspective of health care providers, the potential problems are almost certain to appear more troublesome than Green imagines.
14. Rawls, *Theory of Justice*, pp. 100–101. The principle of redress, as Rawls uses the expression, calls for compensation for "undeserved inequalities" such as the inequalities of birth and natural endowment.
15. For example, queuing may be justified in terms of preserving already established trust relationships, and random selection may be justified in terms of eliminating, so far as possible, the element of human judgment. Neither of these justifications has to do with providing equality of access.

It is also interesting to note that Erikson suggests that the quarrel between those claiming rights on the basis of "getting there first" and those claiming rights because of needs may stem from the sibling rivalry of childhood. "For the former [i.e., bigger or older child] claims a right of ownership based on having been there first and being stronger, the latter [i.e., younger or smaller child] an equal right on the basis of having come last and being weaker—contradictions not easily reconciled either in systems of child training or in political systems." Erik Erikson, *Childhood and Society,* 2d ed. (New York: W. W. Norton, 1963), p. 412.

16. James Childress, "Who Shall Live When Not All Can Live?" *Soundings* XLIII (Winter 1970): 347.
17. Ibid., p. 352.
18. Rawls, *Theory of Justice,* p. 374.
19. Stuart Hinds, "On the Relations of Medical Triage to World Famine: An Historical Survey," in *Lifeboat Ethics: The Moral Dilemmas of World Hunger,* ed. George R. Lucas, Jr. and Thomas W. Ogletree (New York: Harper and Row, 1976), pp. 38–39.
20. Jay Katz and Alexander Morgan Capron, *Catastrophic Diseases: Who Decides What?* (New York: Russell Sage Foundation, 1975), p. 194. The authors make it clear that by "drawing" they mean some computerized system of random number selection.
21. For discussions of random selection as prescribed in ancient Jewish literature see A. M. Hasofer, "Studies in the History of Probability and Statistics: Random Mechanisms in Talmudic Literature," *Biometrika* LIV (1967): 316–321; and Nachem L. Rabinovitch, *Probability and Statistical Inference in Ancient and Medieval Jewish Literature* (Toronto: University of Toronto Press, 1973), especially chap. 2, "Random Mechanisms," pp. 21–35. The authors point out that the Bible prescribes random mechanisms for such diverse practices as the allocation of land among the tribes and families (Numbers 26:55), the assignment of towns to the priests and Levites (I Chronicles 6:39), and military conscription (Judges 20:9–10). Moreover, there is considerable evidence that the ancient sages recognized the need to keep the random process free of biases so that fair opportunity was provided to all. It is also interesting to note that casting lots was sometimes seen as an alternative to queuing. Hasofer refers to the process for selecting the priests who were given the honored responsibility of removing the ashes from the altar. He says: "[I]n older times there used to be a race up the ramp of the Altar, and he that came first within four cubits of the Altar secured the task of clearing the ashes. Only if two of the participants were equal did they use lots. But once it happened that two were equal, and one of them pushed the other so that he fell and his leg was broken; and when the Court saw that they incurred danger, they ordained that they should not clear the Altar save by lots," p. 319. For a brief discussion of the ethics of random selection, see Sid Z.

Leiman, "The Ethics of Lottery," *Kennedy Institute Quarterly Report* IV (Summer 1978): 8–11.

22. Charles Fried, *An Anatomy of Values: Problems of Personal and Social Choice* (Cambridge: Harvard University Press, 1970), pp. 202–203. "My argument is . . . that in many situations in the absence of some explicit arrangement to which all involved parties have consented to be bound, there may be no better approximation to equality than the rough and ready randomization entailed by the principle of letting the loss lie where it falls," p. 203. Fried's illustration is that of shipwreck victims swimming in search of a life-saving plank. His contention is that conducting a lottery would subject the person who arrived first at the plank to a kind of double jeopardy or a "second lottery." Finding the plank first, on this view, is sufficient randomization. But, for reasons already stated, this view loses force in the case of medical triage for a resource such as the artificial heart.

23. Rawls, *Theory of Justice*, p. 6.

24. Ramsey, *Patient as Person*, p. 275.

25. Jacques P. Thiroux, *Ethics: Theory and Practice* (Encino, Cal.: Glencoe Press, 1977), p. 33.

26. Green also makes this application of the difference principle to the delivery of health care. His example is giving physicians priority so that they can be innoculated first if the population is threatened with a plague. In such circumstances, Green suggests that the contrctors might "be prepared to sacrifice some equal access to health care in order to secure such care more firmly in the future." "Health Care and Justice," p. 118.

27. William Frankena, "The Concept of Social Justice," in *Social Justice*, ed. Richard Brandt (Englewood Cliffs: Prentice-Hall, 1962) pp. 15–16.

28. "Scarce Medical Resources," *Columbia Law Review* LXIX (April 1969): 652.

29. See, for example, J. Hyatt, "The Cost of Living: Some Kidney Patients Die for Lack of Funds for Machine Treatment," *Wall Street Journal* 10 March 1969, pp. 1 and 19. The author says that renal dialysis centers had to begin relying more on the patients' ability to pay because federal government funds for research and development had been cut back in an economy drive necessitated by the war in Vietnam. In the case of one Minneapolis center, patients were required to place $12,000 in escrow before treatment could begin.

30. See, for example, David Sanders and Jesse Dukeminier, Jr., "Medical Advance and Legal Lag: Hemodialysis and Kidney Transplantation," *U.C.L.A. Law Review* XV (February 1968): 380. The authors grant that basing triage on the ability to pay is imperfect, but they consider the approach better than allocation based on comparisons of general social value.

31. Katz and Capron, *Catastrophic Diseases*, pp. 185–188.

32. Ibid., pp. 187–188. Later, the authors consider a "wealth distribution neutral market" in which the required payment for the scarce resources would be pegged to the candidates' ability to pay so that the rich would pay more and the poor would pay less. But in addition to such problems as lying about one's financial status and the development of black markets, the authors say: "There is something very unattractive about a governmental agency expending great energy and intellectual resources to be constantly adjusting the price of the treatment for each wealth category . . . so as to be able to announce that 'we have found just the price where enough of you, whether rich or poor, will choose to die rather than avail yourselves of this treatment,'" p. 188. It should also be noted that the various factors involved in the market approach to the distribution of scarce resources have been treated in great detail in Guido Calabresi and Philip Bobbitt, *Tragic Choices: The Conflicts Society Confronts in the Allocation of Tragically Scarce Resources* (New York: W. W. Norton, 1978).

33. *The Totally Implantable Artificial Heart: Economic, Ethical, Legal, Medical, Psychiatric, Social Implications* (Washington, D.C.: Department of Health, Education and Welfare, 1973), p. 148.

34. Benjamin Freedman, "The Case for Medical Care, Inefficient or Not," *Hastings Center Report* VII (April 1977): 33.

35. Nicholas Rescher, "The Allocation of Exotic Medical Lifesaving Therapy," *Ethics* LXXIX (April 1969): 179.

36. W. D. Ross, *The Right and the Good* (Oxford: Clarendon Press, 1973), p. 58. It is interesting to note that Ross omits from the category of justice such acts as the payment of debts and reparations, p. 27. By justice he means only the distribution of benefits in accordance with virtue, pp. 21 and 26. By moral virtue he means "action, or the disposition to act, from any one of certain motives, of which at all events the most notable are the desire to do one's duty, the desire to bring into being something that is good, and the desire to give pleasure to save pain to others," p. 134.

37. For example, the labor leader on the Seattle committee for the selection of renal dialysis patients said: "That's why knowing about a candidate's past life would rate so heavily with me—it's an indication of *character.*" Shana Alexander, "They Decide Who Lives, Who Dies: Medical Miracle Puts a Moral Burden on a Small Committee," *Life* 9 November 1962, p. 123. The context of this statement indicates that at least part of the committee member's concern stemmed from a desire to achieve maximum efficiency; people of good character were thought to be better treatment risks. However, it is also obvious that moral character *per se* was a consideration in the decision making process as was evidenced by the rejection of prostitutes and criminals.

38. On this point see David Miller, *Social Justice* (Oxford: Clarendon Press, 1976), pp. 96 ff.
39. Ibid., p. 85.
40. Rawls, *Theory of Justice*, pp. 103–104.
41. Ibid., p. 15.
42. Ibid., p. 310.
43. It is not surprising, for example, that Robert Nozick finds Rawls's position on merit to be incredible. According to Nozick, "This line of argument can succeed in blocking the introduction of a person's autonomous choices and actions (and their results) only by attributing *everything* noteworthy about the person completely to certain sorts of 'external' factors. So denigrating a person's autonomy and prime responsibility for his actions is a risky line to take for a theory that otherwise wishes to buttress the dignity and self-respect of autonomous beings . . . " *Anarchy, State, and Utopia* (New York: Basic Books, 1974), p. 214. It is interesting to note, on the other hand, that some of Rawls's most severe critics consider his treatment of merit to be one of the few bright spots in Rawls's work. See, for example, Brian Barry, *The Liberal Theory of Justice* (Oxford: Clarendon Press, 1973), pp. 155–156.
44. On this point see Gene Outka, "Social Justice and Equal Access to Health Care," in *Love and Society*, ed. James Johnson and David Smith (Missoula: Scholars Press, 1974), pp. 189–193.
45. Isaiah 32:17.
46. Michael Novak, "The Social World of Individuals," *Hastings Center Studies II (September 1974): 42.*

Selected Bibliography

Ethical Theory

Anscombe, G. E. M. "Who Is Wronged?" *The Oxford Review* V (1967): 16–17.

Aristotle. *Nichomachean Ethics*. Translated by Martin Ostwald. Indianapolis: Bobbs-Merrill Company, 1962.

Arrow, Kenneth J. "Some Ordinalist-Utilitarian Notes on Rawls's Theory of Justice." *The Journal of Philosophy* LXX (May 10, 1973), 245–263.

Baier, Kurt. *The Moral Point of View: A Rational Basis of Ethics*. New York: Random House, 1965.

Barry, Brian. *The Liberal Theory of Justice: A Critical Examination of the Principal Doctrines in 'A Theory of Justice' by John Rawls*. Oxford: Clarendon Press, 1973.

———. "On Social Justice." *The Oxford Review* V (1967): 29–52.

Bayles, Michael D. "The Price of Life." *Ethics* LXXXIX (October (1978): 20–34.

Benn, Stanley I. "Egalitarianism and the Equal Consideration of Interests." *Justice and Equality*. Edited by Hugo A. Bedau. Englewood Cliffs, N.J.: Prentice-Hall, 1971.

Blocker, H. Gene, and Smith, E. H. *John Rawls' Theory of Social Justice*. Athens: Ohio University Press, 1979.

Bowie, Norman E. *Towards a New Theory of Distributive Justice*. Amherst: University of Massachusetts Press, 1971.

Brandt, R. B. *Ethical Theory: The Problems of Normative and Critical Ethics*. Englewood Cliffs: Prentice-Hall, 1959.

———. *A Theory of the Good and the Right*. New York: Oxford University Press, 1979.

Brandt, R. B., ed. *Social Justice*. Englewood Cliffs: Prentice-Hall, 1962.

Broad, C. D. *Five Types of Ethical Theory*. London: Routledge and Kegan Paul, 1930.

Brunner, Emil. *Justice and the Social Order*. Translated by Mary Hottinger. New York: Harper and Brothers, 1945.

Cahn, Edmond. *The Moral Decision: Right and Wrong in the Light of American Law*. Bloomington: Indiana University Press, 1955.

————. *The Sense of Injustice.* Bloomington: Indiana University Press, 1949.

Callahan, Daniel. *The Tyranny of Survival: And Other Pathologies of Civilized Life.* New York: Macmillan Publishing Company, 1973.

Childress, James F. "The Identification of Ethical Principles." *The Journal of Religious Ethics* V (Spring 1977): 39–66.

Choptiany, Leonard. "A Critique of John Rawls's Principles of Justice." *Ethics* LXXXVIII (1973): 146–150.

Clark, Henry B. "Justice as Fairness and Christian Ethics." *Soundings* LVI (1973): 359–369.

Daniels, Norman, ed. *Reading Rawls: Critical Studies of "A Theory of Justice."* New York: Basic Books, 1976.

Daube, David. *Collaboration with Tyranny in Rabbinic Law.* London: Oxford University Press, 1965.

Davis, Henry, S.J. *Human Acts, Law, Sin, Virtue.* Vol. I of *Moral and Pastoral Theology.* New York: Sheed and Ward, 1946.

Donagan, Alan. *The Theory of Morality.* Chicago: University of Chicago Press, 1977.

Downie, R. S., and Telfer, Elizabeth. *Respect for Persons.* New York: Schocken Books, 1970.

Dworkin, Ronald. "The Original Position." *Reading Rawls: Critical Studies on Rawls' "A Theory of Justice."* Edited by Norman Daniels. New York: Basic Books, 1976.

Dyck, Arthur J. *On Human Care: An Introduction to Ethics.* Nashville: Abingdon, 1977.

Feinberg, Joel. "Duty and Obligation in the Non-Ideal World." *The Journal of Philosophy* LXX (May 10, 1973): 263–275.

Finnin, William M., Jr., and Smith, Gerald A. *The Morality of Scarcity: Limited Resources and Social Policy.* Baton Rouge: Louisiana State University Press, 1979.

Firth, Roderick. "Ethical Absolutism and the Ideal Observer." *Philosophy and Phenomenological Research* XII (1952).

Frankena, William K. "The Concept of Social Justice." *Social Justice.* Edited by Richard B. Brandt. Englewood Cliffs: Prentice-Hall, 1962.

————.*Ethics.* 2d ed. Englewood Cliffs: Prentice-Hall, 1973.

Fried, Charles. *An Anatomy of Values.* Cambridge: Harvard University Press, 1970.

————. "Natural Law and the Concept of Justice." *Ethics* LXXIV (July 1964): 237–254.

————. "Reason and Action." *Natural Law Forum* XI (1966): 13–35.

Fuller, Lon L. "The Case of the Speluncean Explorers." *Harvard Law Review* LXII (1949): 616–645.

Gustafson, James. *Can Ethics Be Christian?* Chicago: University of Chicago Press, 1975.

Hardin, Garrett. *Exploring New Ethics for Survival.* New York: Viking Press, 1972.

———. "Living on a Lifeboat." *BioScience* XXIV (October 1974): 561–568.

Hare, R. M. *Freedom and Reason*. London: Oxford University Press, 1963.

———. *The Language of Morals*. London: Oxford University Press, 1964.

———. "Rawls' Theory of Justice." *Reading Rawls: Critical Studies on Rawls' "A Theory of Justice."* Edited by Norman Daniels. New York: Basic Books, 1976.

Hart, H. L. A. "Are There Any Natural Rights? *Philosophical Review* LXIV (1955): 175–191.

———. *The Concept of Law*. Oxford: Clarendon Press, 1961.

Hauerwas, Stanley. "Natural Law, Tragedy, and Theological Ethics." *The American Journal of Jurisprudence* XX (1975): 1–19.

Heilbroner, Robert L. *An Inquiry into the Human Prospect*. New York: W. W. Norton and Company, 1974.

Honderich, Ted. "The Use of the Basic Proposition of *A Theory of Justice.*" *Mind* LXXXIV (1975): 63–78.

Hubin, D. Clayton. "The Scope of Justice." *Philosophy and Public Affairs* IX (Fall 1979): 3–24.

Hume, David. *Enquiries Concerning Human Understanding and Concerning the Principles of Morals*. Edited by L. A. Selby-Bigge. 3d ed. Oxford: Clarendon Press, 1975.

———. *Hume's Ethical Writings*. Edited by Alasdair MacIntyre. London: Collier Books, 1965.

Jonas, Hans. "Technology and Responsibility: Reflections on the New Tasks of Ethics." *Religion and the Humanizing of Man*. Edited by James M. Robinson. Riverside, Ca.: Riverside Color Press, 1972.

Kant, Immanuel. *Groundwork of the Metaphysic of Morals*. Translated by H. J. Paton. New York: Harper and Row, 1964.

———. *The Doctrine of Virtue*. Part II of *The Metaphysic of Morals*. Translated by M. J. Gregor. New York: Harper and Row, 1964.

Kaufmann, Walter. *Without Guilt and Justice: From Decidophobia to Autonomy*. New York: Peter H. Wyden, 1973.

Kelbley, Charles A., ed. *The Value of Justice*. Bronx, N.Y.: Fordham University Press, 1979.

Leiman, Sid Z. "The Ethics of Lottery." *The Kennedy Institute Quarterly Report* IV (Summer 1978): 8–11.

———. "The Sinking of the William Brown: A Case Study in Jewish Ethics." Unpublished paper, 1975.

Lucas, J. R. *On Justice*. New York: Oxford University Press, 1980.

Lyons, Davis. *Forms and Limits of Utilitarianism*. Oxford: Clarendon Press, 1965.

———. "Nature and Soundness of the Contract and Coherence Arguments." *Reading Rawls: Critical Studies on Rawls' "A Theory of Justice."* Edited by Norman Daniels. New York: Basic Books, 1976.

———. "Review of Nicholas Rescher: *Distributive Justice: A Constructive Critique of the Utilitarian Theory of Distribution.*" *Philosophical Review* LXXVIII (1969): 265–268.

McCoy, Thomas R. "Comment on John Rawls' *A Theory of Justice.*" *Soundings* LVI (1973): 349–358.

Mill, John Stuart. *Utilitarianism.* Edited by Samuel Gorovitz. New York: Bobbs-Merrill Company, 1971.

Miller, David. *Social Justice.* Oxford: Clarendon Press, 1976.

Nagel, Thomas. "Libertarianism without Foundations." Review of *Anarchy, State, and Utopia,* by Robert Nozick. *The Yale Law Journal* LXXXV (1975): 136–149.

———. "Rawls on Justice." *Reading Rawls: Critical Studies on Rawls' "A Theory of Justice."* Edited by Norman Daniels. New York: Basic Books, 1976.

Niebuhr, Reinhold. *Human Destiny.* Vol. II of *The Nature and Destiny of Man.* New York: Charles Scribners' Sons, 1943.

Novak, Michael. "The Social World of Individuals." *Hastings Center Studies* II (1974): 37–44.

Nozick, Robert. *Anarchy, State and Utopia.* New York: Basic Books, 1974.

Peffer, Rodney. "A Defense of Rights to Well-Being." *Philosophy and Public Affairs* VIII (Fall 1978): 64–87.

Perelman, Chaim. *The Idea of Justice and the Problem of Argument.* Translated by J. Petrie. London: Routledge and Kegan Paul, 1963.

Ramsey, Paul. *Basic Christian Ethics.* New York: Charles Scribners' Sons, 1950.

———. *Nine Modern Moralists.* Englewood Cliffs: Prentice-Hall, 1962.

Raphael, D. D. "Critical Notice, *A Theory of Justice.*" *Mind* LXXXIII (1974): 118–127.

Rawls, John. *A Theory of Justice.* Cambridge: Harvard University Press, 1971.

Rempel, Henry David. "Justice as Efficiency." *Ethics* LXXIX (January 1969): 150–156.

Rescher, Nicholas. *Distributive Justice: A Constructive Critique of the Utilitarian Theory of Distribution.* New York: Bobbs-Merrill Company, 1966.

Ross, W. D. *The Right and the Good.* Oxford: Clarendon Press, 1973.

Ryan, John A. *Distributive Justice.* New York: Macmillan Company, 1942.

Schroeder, Donald N. "John Rawls and Contract Theory." *Soundings* LVI (1973): 338–348.

Sidgwick, Henry. *The Methods of Ethics.* 7th ed. New York: Dover Publications, 1966.

Sterba, James P. *The Demands of Justice.* Notre Dame: University of Notre Dame Press, 1980.

Teitelman, Michael. "The Limits of Individualism" *The Journal of Philosophy* LXIX (October 5, 1972): 545–556.

Toulmin, Stephen. *An Examination of the Place of Reason in Ethics.* New York: Cambridge University Press, 1950.

Tracy, David. *A Blessed Rage for Order.* New York: Seabury, 1975.

Vlastos, Gregory. "Justice and Equality." *Social Justice.* Edited by Richard B. Brandt. Englewood Cliffs: Prentice-Hall, 1962.

Walsh, Vivian C. *Scarcity and Evil.* Englewood Cliffs: Prentice-Hall, 1961.

Warnock, G. J. *Contemporary Moral Philosophy.* London: Macmillan and Company, 1967.

Williams, Bernard A. O. "The Idea of Equality." *Justice and Equality.* Edited by Hugo A. Bedau. Englewood Cliffs: Prentice-Hall, 1971.

Wogaman, J. Philip. *A Christian Method of Moral Judgment.* Philadelphia: Westminster Press, 1976.

Wolff, Robert Paul. *Understanding Rawls: A Reconstruction and Critique of "A Theory of Justice."* Princeton: Princeton University Press, 1977.

Medical Ethics

American Friends Service Committee. *Who Shall Live? Man's Control Over Birth and Death.* New York: Hill and Wang, 1970.

Annas, George J. "Allocation of Artificial Hearts in the Year 2002: 'Minerva v. National Health Agency.'" *American Journal of Law and Medicine* III (Spring 1977): 59–76.

Basson, Marc D. "Choosing among Candidates for Scarce Medical Resources." *The Journal of Medicine and Philosophy* IV (September 1979): 313–333.

Bauer, K. H. "Über Rechtsfragen bei homologer Organstransplantation aus der Sich des Klinikers." *Der Chirurg* XXXVIII (June 1967): 245–251.

Boyd, Kenneth M., ed. *The Ethics of Resource Allocation in Health Care.* Edinburgh: Edinburgh University Press, 1979.

Branson, Roy. "Justice and Health Care." *The Encyclopedia of Bioethics.* Edited by Warren T. Reich. New York: Free Press, 1978.

Bryant, John H. "Principles of Justice as a Basis for Conceptualizing a Health Care System." *International Journal of Health Services* VII (1977): 707–719, 721–739.

Camenisch, Paul R. "The Right to Health Care: A Contractual Approach." *Soundings* LXII (Fall 1979): 293–310.

Campbell, Alastair V. *Medicine, Health and Justice: The Problem of Priorities.* Edinburgh: Churchill Livingstone, 1978.

––––––. *Moral Dilemmas in Medicine.* London: Churchill Livingstone, 1972.

Childress, James. "Priorities in the Allocation of Health Care Resources. *Soundings* LXII (Fall 1979): 256–274.

———. "Rationing of Medical Treatment." *The Encyclopedia of Bioethics*. Edited by Warren T. Reich. New York: Free Press, 1978.

———. "Who Shall Live When Not All Can Live?" *Soundings*, XLIII (1970): 339–362.

Committee on Ethics of the American Heart Association. "Ethical Considerations of the Left Ventricular Assist Device." *Journal of the American Medical Association* CCXXXV (February 1976): 823–824.

Curran, Charles E. *Politics, Medicine, and Christian Ethics: A Dialogue with Paul Ramsey*. Philadelphia: Fortress Press, 1973.

Cutler, D. R., ed. *Updating Life and Death: Essays in Ethics and Medicine*. Boston: Beacon Press, 1968.

Daniels, Norman. "Rights to Health Care and Distributive Justice: Programmatic Worries." *The Journal of Medicine and Philosophy* IV (1979): 174–191.

Del Guercio, Louis R. M. "Triage in Cold Blood." *Critical Care Medicine* V (July-August 1977): 167–169.

"Due Process in the Allocation of Scarce Lifesaving Medical Resources." *The Yale Law Journal* LXXXIV (July 1975): 1734–1749.

Duncan, A. S. "Scientific and Technological Development in Biology and Medicine which May Lead to the Infringement of Human Rights." *Protection of Human Rights in the Light of Scientific and Technological Progress in Biology and Medicine*. Geneva: World Health Organization, 1974.

Dyck, Arthur J. "Ethics and Medicine." *Linacre Quarterly* XL (August 1973): 182–200.

Englehardt, H. Tristram. "Personal Health Care or Preventive Care: Distributing Scarce Medical Resources." *Soundings* LXIII (Fall 1980): 234–256.

Fellner, Carl H. "Organ Donation: For Whose Sake?" *Annals of Internal Medicine* LXXIX (October 1973): 589–592.

Fletcher, Joseph F. "Donor Nephrectomies and Moral Responsibility." *Journal of the American Medical Women's Association* XXIII (December 1968): 1085–1091.

———. *The Greatest Good of the Greatest Number: A New Frontier in the Morality of Medical Care*. Sanger Lecture, no. 7. Richmond: Medical College of Virginia Foundation, 1971.

Foot, Philippa. "The Problem of Abortion and the Doctrine of the Double Effect." *The Oxford Review* V (1967): 5–15.

Freedman, Benjamin. "The Case for Medical Care, Inefficient or Not." *The Hastings Center Report* VII (April 1977): 31–39.

Freund, Paul A., ed. *Experimentation with Human Subjects*. New York: George Braziller, 1970.

Fried, Charles. "Equality and Rights in Medical Care." *The Hastings Center Report* VI (February 1976): 29–34.

──────. *Medical Experimentation: Personal Integrity and Social Policy.* New York: American Elsevier Publishing Company, 1974.

──────. "Rights and Health Care—Beyond Equity and Efficiency." *The New England Journal of Medicine* CCXCIII (July 31, 1975): 241–245.

Glover, Jonathan. *Causing Death and Saving Lives.* New York: Penguin Books, 1977.

Gorovitz, Samuel. "Ethics and the Allocation of Medical Resources." *Medical Research Engineering* V (1966): 5–7.

Green, Ronald M. "Health Care and Justice in Contract Theory Perspective." *Ethics and Health Policy.* Edited by Robert M. Veatch and Roy Branson. Cambridge, Mass.: Ballinger Publishing Company, 1976.

Gustafson, James M. "Basic Ethical Issues in Biomedical Fields." *Soundings* LIII (Summer 1970): 151–180.

Hiatt, Howard H. "Protecting the Medical Commons: Who is Responsible." *The New England Journal of Medicine* CCXCIII (July 31, 1975): 235–241.

Illich, Ivan. *Medical Nemesis.* New York: Pantheon Books, 1976.

Jakobovits, Immanuel. *Jewish Medical Ethics: A Comparative and Historical Study of the Jewish Religious Attitude to Medicine and its Practice.* New York: Bloch Publishing Company, 1975.

Jonas, Hans. "Philosophical Reflections on Experimenting with Human Subjects." *Experimentation with Human Subjects.* Edited by Paul A. Freund. New York: George Braziller, 1970.

Jonsen, Albert R. "A New Ethic for Medicine?" *The Western Journal of Medicine* CXX (February 1974): 169–173.

──────. "Sounding Board: Scientific Medicine and Therapeutic Choice." *The New England Journal of Medicine* CCXCII (May 22, 1975): 1126–1127.

──────. "The Totally Implantable Artificial Heart." *The Hastings Center Report* III (November 1973): 1–4.

Jonsen, Albert R., and Butler, Lewis H. "Public Ethics and Policy Making." *The Hastings Center Report* V (August 1974): 19–31.

Jonsen, Albert R., and Hellegers, Andre E. "Conceptual Foundations for an Ethics of Medical Care." *Ethics of Health Care.* Edited by Laurence R. Tancredi. Washington, D.C.: National Academy of Sciences, 1974.

Jonsen, Albert R., and Jameton, Andrew L. "Social and Political Responsibilities of Physicians." *The Journal of Medicine and Philosophy* II (December 1977): 376–400.

Jonsen, Albert R. et al. "Critical Issues in Newborn Intensive Care: A Conference Report and Policy Proposal." *Pediatrics* LV (June 6, 1975): 756–768.

Kass, Leon R. "The New Biology: What Price Relieving Man's Estate? *Science* CLXXIV (November 19, 1971): 779–788.

Katz, Jay, and Capron, Alexander M. *Catastrophic Diseases: Who Decides What?* New York: Russell Sage Foundation, 1975.

Bibliography

King, Maurice. "Personal Health Care: The Quest for a Human Right." *Human Rights in Health: Ciba Symposium 23.* New York: Associated Scientific Publishers, 1974.

Leach, Gerald. *The Biocrats: Implications of Medical Progress.* Revised ed. Baltimore: Penguin Books, 1970.

Lebacqz, Karen A. "Prenatal Diagnosis: Distributive Justice and the Quality of Life." Ph.D. dissertation, Harvard University, 1974.

Livingston, Gordon S. "Medicine and the Military." *Humanistic Perspectives in Medical Ethics.* Edited by Maurice B. Visscher. Buffalo: Prometheus Books, 1972.

Lucas, George R., Jr., ed. *Triage in Medicine and Society.* Vol. III: *Inquiries in Medical Ethics.* Houston: Institute of Religion and Human Development, 1975.

McCormick, Richard. "To Save or Let Die: The Dilemma of Modern Medicine." *Journal of the American Medical Association* CCXXIX (July 8, 1974): 172–176.

Masters, Roger D. "Is Contract an Adequate Basis for Medical Ethics?" *The Hastings Center Report* V (December 1975): 24–28.

Mechanic, David. "Rationing Medical Care." *The Center Magazine* XI (September-October 1978): 22–31.

――――. "Rationing Health Care: Public Policy and the Medical Marketplace." *The Hastings Center Report* VI (February 1976): 34–37.

"A New Ethic for Medicine and Society." *California Medicine* CXIII (September 1970): 67–68.

O'Donnell, Thomas. "The Morality of Triage." *Georgetown Medical Bulletin* XIV (August 1960): 68–71.

Outka, Gene. "Social Justice and Equal Access to Health Care." *The Journal of Religious Ethics* II (Spring 1973): 11–32.

"Patient Selection for Artificial and Transplanted Organs." *Harvard Law Review* LXXXII (1969): 1322–1342.

Pellegrino, Edmund D. "Medical Morality and Medical Economics." *The Hastings Center Report* VIII (August 1978): 8–12.

Percival, Thomas. *Medical Ethics.* Edited by Chauncey D. Leake. New York: Robert E. Krieger, 1975. [Note: This is a reprint of the 1927 edition published by Williams and Wilkins, Baltimore.]

Protection of Human Rights in the Light of Scientific and Technological Progress in Biology and Medicine. Geneva: World Health Organization, 1974.

Pulvertaft, R. J. V. "The Individual and the Group in Modern Medicine." *The Lancet* II (November 1, 1952): 839–842.

Ramsey, Paul. *The Patient as Person.* New Haven: Yale University Press, 1970.

Rescher, Nicholas. "The Allocation of Exotic Medical Lifesaving Therapy." *Ethics* LXXIX (April 1969): 173–186.

――――. "Ethical Issues Regarding the Delivery of Health-Care Services." *Connecticut Medicine* XLI (August 1977): 501–506.

Sanders, David, and Dukeminier, Jesse, Jr. "Medical Advance and Legal Lag: Hemodialysis and Kidney Transplantation." *U.C.L.A. Law Review* XV (February 1968): 357–413.

"Scarce Medical Resources." *Columbia Law Review* LXIX (April 1969): 620–692.

Schiffer, R. M., and Freedman, Benjamin. "Case Studies in Bioethics: The Last Bed in the ICU." *The Hastings Center Report* VII (December 1977): 21–22.

Schreiner, G. E. "Problems of Ethics in Relation to Haemodialysis and Transplantation." *Ethics in Medical Progress.* Edited by G. E. W. Wolstenholme. Boston: Little, Brown and Company, 1966.

Shapiro, Michael H. "Who Merits Merit? Problems in Distributive Justice and Utility Posed by the New Biology." *Southern California Law Review* XLVIII (November 1974): 318–370.

Shatin, Leo. "Medical Care and the Social Worth of a Man." *American Journal of Orthopsychiatry* XXVI (1966): 96–101.

Telfer, Elizabeth. "Justice, Welfare and Health Care." *Journal of Medical Ethics* II (1976): 107–111.

Thielicke, Helmut. "The Doctor as Judge of Who Shall Live and Who Shall Die." *Who Shall Live?* Edited by Kenneth Vaux. Philadelphia: Fortress Press, 1970.

Titmuss, Richard. *The Gift Relationship.* New York: Vintage Books, 1971.

United Nations Economic and Social Council, Commission on Human Rights. "Developments in Medicine." Part II of *Human Rights and Scientific and Technological Developments.* Memeographed. Geneva, 1975.

Vaux, Kenneth. *Who Shall Live?* Philadelphia: Fortress Press, 1970.

Veatch, Robert M. "Models for Ethical Medicine in a Revolutionary Age." *The Hastings Center Report,* II (June 1972): 5–7.

Veatch, Robert M., and Branson, Roy. *Ethics and Health Policy.* Cambridge, Mass.: Ballinger Publishing Company, 1976.

Waitzkin, Howard B., and Waterman, Barbara. *The Exploitation of Illness in a Capitalist Society.* New York: Bobbs-Merrill Company, 1974.

Westervelt, Frederic B. "A Reply to Childress: The Selection Process as Viewed from Within." *Soundings* XLVIII (Winter 1970): 356–362.

Wolstenholme, G. E. W., ed. *Ethics in Medical Progress: With Special Reference to Transplantation.* Boston: Little, Brown and Company, 1966.

Young, Robert. "Some Criteria for Making Decisions Concerning the Distribution of Scarce Medical Resources." *Theory and Decision* VI (1975): 439–455.

Military Medicine

Bainbridge, W. S. *Report on Medical and Surgical Developments of the War.* Washington, D.C.: United States Government Printing Office, 1919.

Beebe, Gilbert W., and DeBakey, Michael E. *Battle Casualties: Incidence, Mortality, and Logistic Considerations.* Springfield: Charles C. Thomas, 1952.

Crile, G. W. "Summarized Report of the Conference on Surgery in Battle Areas." *War Medicine* II (October 1918): 299.

Fulton, J. F. "Medicine, Warfare, and History." *Journal of the American Medical Association* CLIII (October 3, 1953): 482-488.

Gross, S. D. *A Manual of Military Surgery, or Hints on the Emergencies of Field, Camp, and Hospital Practice.* Philadelphia: J. B. Lippincott and Company, 1862.

Handbook of the Hospital Corps: United States Navy. Washington, D.C.: United States Government Printing Office, 1959.

Hennen, John. *Principles of Military Surgery.* Philadelphia: Carey and Lea, 1830.

Hinds, Stuart W. "On the Relations of Medical Triage to World Famine: An Historical Survey." *Lifeboat Ethics.* Edited by George R. Lucas, Jr. and Thomas W. Ogletree. New York: Harper and Row, 1976.

History of the American Field Service in France, 1914-1917. Boston: Houghton Mifflin, 1920.

Keefer, Chester. "Penicillin: A Wartime Achievement in Military Medicine." *Advances in Military Medicine.* Edited by E. C. Andrus. Boston: Little, Brown and Company, 1948.

Keen, W. W. *The Treatment of War Wounds.* Philadelphia: W. B. Saunders Company, 1917.

Laffin, John. *Surgeons in the Field.* London: Aldine Press, 1970.

Larrey, D. J. *Surgical Memoirs of the Campaigns of Russia, Germany, and France.* Translated by John C. Mercer. Philadelphia: Carey and Lea, 1832.

Lee, Roger I. "The Case for the More Efficient Treatment of Light Casualties in Military Hospitals." *The Military Surgeon* XLII (March 1918): 283-285.

Lueth, Harold. "Streamlining Military Medical Care." *Hygeia* XXI (March 1943): 194-195.

Medical Service Theater of Operations, Field Manual FM 8-10. Washington, D.C.: United States Department of the Army, 1959.

Military Medical Manual. 6th ed. Harrisburg: The Military Service Publishing Company, 1945.

Poynter, F. N. L., ed. *Medicine and Surgery in the Great War (1914-1918).* London: The Wellcome Institute of the History of Medicine, 1968.

Richardson, Robert G. *Larrey: Surgeon to Napoleon's Imperial Guard.* London: John Murray, 1974.

Ritter, A. "Triage." *Vierteljahrsschrift für Schweizerische Sanitätsoffiziere* XXII (1945): 8–18.

Snyder, Howard E. "Problems of Triage and Evacuation." Symposium on the Treatment of Trauma in the Armed Forces, 10–12 March 1952. Washington, D.C.: Army Medical Service Graduate School, 1952.

Straub, Paul F. *Medical Service in Campaign: A Handbook for Medical Officers in the Field.* Philadelphia: P. Blakiston's Son and Company, 1910.

Stromeyer, L. *Maximen der Kriegsheilkunst.* Hannover: Hahn'sche Hofbuchhandlung, 1855.

"The Tale of a Casualty Clearing Station." *Blackwood's Edinburgh Magazine* CC (November 1916): 610–640 ff.

Tidy, Henry L., ed. *Inter-Allied Conferences on War Medicine, 1942–1945.* New York: Staples Press, 1947.

Trueta, Jose. *Principles and Practice of War Surgery.* St. Louis: C. V. Mosby, 1943.

Tuttle, A. D. *Handbook for the Medical Soldier.* New York: William Wood and Company, 1927.

United States Department of Defense. *Emergency War Surgery.* Washington, D.C.: United States Government Printing Office, 1975.

Von Greyerz, Waldo. *Psychology of Survival: Human Reactions to the Catastrophes of War.* New York: Elsevier Publishing Company, 1962.

Wallace, Cuthbert, and Fraser, John. *Surgery at a Casualty Clearing Station.* London: A. and C. Black, Ltd., 1918.

Warren, Richard, and Jackson, James H. "Suggestions for First-Aid Treatment of Casualties from Atomic Bombing." *The New England Journal of Medicine* CCXLIII (November 2, 1950): 696–698.

Whitman, Walt. *The Wound Dresser: Letters Written to His Mother from the Hospitals in Washington During the Civil War.* Edited by R. M. Bucke. New York: The Bodley Press, 1949.

———. "Wounds and Diseases." *Complete Prose Works.* New York: Appleton and Company, 1910.

Woods, Hutchinson. *The Doctor in War.* Boston: Houghton Mifflin Company, 1918.

Disaster and Emergency Medicine

Baker, George and Chapman, Dwight, eds. *Man and Society in Disaster.* New York: Basic Books, 1962.

Byrn, Katherine. "Disaster Brings out the Best in People." *Science Digest* LXXIV (August 1973): 29–34.

Bibliography

Chayet, Neil L. "Medical Care in a Disaster." *Legal Implications of Emergency Care*. New York: Appleton-Century-Crofts, 1969.

Dressler, Donald P., et al. "The Physician and Mass Casualty Care." *The Journal of Trauma* XI (March 1971): 260-262.

Fairley, James. "Mass Disaster Schemes." *British Medical Journal* IV (November 29, 1969): 551-553.

Gierson, Eugene D., and Richman, Leon S. "Valley Triage: An Approach to Mass Casualty Care." *The Journal of Trauma* XV (March 1975): 193-196.

Koughan, Martin. "Goodbye, San Francisco: Measuring the Effect of the Inevitable Earthquake." *Harper's Magazine*, September 1975, pp. 30-36.

McLeod, Kathryn A. "Learning to Take the Trauma of Triage." *RN* XXXVIII (July 1975): 23-27.

Office of Emergency Services, City and County of San Francisco. "Emergency Medical Care: General Operational Procedures." Mimeographed. San Francisco, March, 1976.

──────. "Emergency Operations Plan." Mimeographed. San Francisco, March 1976.

──────. "San Francisco Earthquake Response Plan." Mimeographed. San Francisco, September 1974.

Sorokin, Pitirim A. *Man and Society in Calamity: The Effects of War, Revolution, Famine, Pestilence Upon Human Mind, Behavior, Social Organization and Cultural Life*. New York: E. P. Dutton and Company, 1942.

Vickery, Donald M. *Triage: Problem-Oriented Sorting of Patients*. Bowie, Md.: Robert J. Brady, 1975.

<hr>

Scarce Medical Resources

Abram, Harry S., and Wadlington, Walter. "Selections of Patients for Artificial and Transplanted Organs." *Annals of Internal Medicine* LXIX (September 1968): 615-620.

Alexander, Shana. "They Decide Who Lives, Who Dies: Medical Miracle Puts a Moral Burden on a Small Committee." *Life*, 9 November 1962, pp. 102 ff.

Altman, Lawrence, K. "Artificial Kidney Use Poses Awesome Questions." *New York Times*, 24 October 1971.

──────. "Costs of Kidney Therapy: Two Fundamental Questions Raised." *New York Times*, 23 January 1973.

Beecher, Henry. "Scarce Resources and Medical Advancement." *Experimentation with Human Subjects*. Edited by Paul Freund. New York: George Braziller, 1969.

Brent, L., ed. "The Shortage of Organs for Clinical Transplantation: Document for Discussion." *British Medical Journal* IV (February 1, 1975): 251–255.

Calne, R. Y. et al. "Shortage of Organs for Transplantation." *British Medical Journal* IV (December 20, 1975).

Cardiology Advisory Committee of the National Heart, Lung and Blood Institute. "Mechanically Assisted Circulation—The Status of the NHLBI Program and Recommendations for the Future." *Artificial Organs* I (November 1977): 39–58.

Cochrane, A. L. *Effectiveness and Efficiency: Random Reflections on Health Services*. London: The Nuffield Provincial Hospital Trust, 1972.

Cooper, Michael H. *Rationing Health Care*. London: Halsted Press, 1975.

Friedman, E. A., and Kountz, S. L. "Impact of HR-1 on the Therapy of End-Stage Uremia." *The New England Journal of Medicine* CCXXVIII (June 14, 1973): 1287.

Hall, C. W. et al. *Artificial Heart: Present and Future*. Washington, D.C.: United States Government Printing Office, 1966.

Hyatt, J. "The Cost of Living: Some Kidney Patients Die for Lack of Funds for Machine Treatment." *Wall Street Journal*, 10 March 1969, pp. 1 and 19.

Jones, Marion, and Jones, Bruce P. "The Allocation of Resources in Production and Distribution of Medical Services in Australia." *The Medical Journal of Australia* I (April 19, 1975): 508–510.

Katz, A. H., and Proctor, D. M. "Social-Psychological Characteristics of Patients Receiving Hemodialysis Treatment for Chronic Renal Failure." Mimeographed. July, 1969.

Kolff, W. J., and Lawson, J. "Perspectives for the Total Artificial Heart." *Transplantation Proceedings* XI (March 1979): 317–324.

Lawson, J., and Kolff, W. J. "The Artificial Heart: Current Status and Clinical Prospects." *Practical Cardiology* V (July 1979): 95–103.

"Long-Term Dialysis Programs: New Selection Criteria, New Problems." *The Hastings Center Report* VI (June 1976): 8–13.

Moore, G. L. "Who Should Be Dialyzed?" *American Journal of Psychiatry* CXXVII (1971): 1208–1209.

Rettig, Richard A. *Health Care Technology: Lessons Learned from the End-Stage Renal Disease Experience*. Santa Monica: Rand Corporation, 1976.

Rettig, Richard A., and Webster, Thomas. *Implementation of the End-Stage Renal Disease Program: A Mixed Pattern of Subsidizing and Regulating the Delivery of Medical Services*. Santa Monica: Rand Corporation, 1975.

Sullivan, Paul et al. "Artificial Internal Organs: Promise, Profits, and Problems," Mimeographed. Harvard Business School, 1966.

"The Totally Implantable Artificial Heart." A Report by the Artificial

Heart Assessment Panel, National Heart and Lung Institute. June 1973.

Unger, Felix. *Assisted Circulation*. New York: Springer-Verlag, 1979.

"Waiting-Lists Lengthen." *The Lancet* I (January 15, 1977): 152.

Miscellany

Acton, Jan P. *Measuring the Monetary Value of Lifesaving Programs*. Santa Monica: Rand Corporation, 1976.

Calabresi, Guido, and Bobbitt, Philip. *Tragic Choices: The Conflicts Society Confronts in the Allocation of Tragically Scarce Resources*. New York: W. W. Norton and Company, 1978.

Court, W. H. B. *Scarcity and Choice in History*. London: Edward Arnold, Ltd., 1970.

Ehrlich, Paul R., and Ehrlich, Anne H. *The End of Affluence*. New York: Ballantine Books, 1974.

Fox, Renee C. *Experiment Perilous*. Glencoe, Ill.: Free Press, 1959.

_____. "A Sociological Perspective on Organ Transplantation and Hemodialysis." *Annals of the New York Academy of Science* CLXIX (1970): 406–428.

Fox, Renee C., and Swazey, Judith P. *The Courage to Fail: A Social View of Organ Transplants and Dialysis*. Chicago: University of Chicago Press, 1974.

Fuchs, Victor R. *Who Shall Live? Health, Economics, and Social Choice*. New York: Basic Books, 1974.

Green, Wade. "Triage." *The New York Times Magazine*. 5 January 1975, pp. 111–122.

Hasofer, A. M. "Studies in the History of Probability and Statistics: Random Mechanisms in Talmudic Literature." *Biometrika* LIV (1967): 316–321.

Jones-Lee, M. W. *The Value of Life: An Economic Analysis*. Chicago: University of Chicago Press, 1976.

Joy, Robert J. T. "Triage—Who is Sorted and Why?" *Hard Choices*. Edited by William Bennett and Barbara Gale. Seattle: KCTS/9 and the University of Washington, 1980.

Knowles, John H., ed. *Doing Better and Feeling Worse: Health in the United States*. New York: W. W. Norton and Company, 1977.

Lewin, Leonard. *Triage*. New York: Dial Press, 1972.

Luce, R. Duncan, and Raiffa, Howard. *Games and Decisions: Introduction and Critical Survey*. New York: Wiley, 1957.

Mooney, Gavid H. *The Valuation of Human Life*. London: Macmillan Press, Ltd., 1977.

Newhouse, Joseph P., and Goldberg, George A. *Allocation of Resources in Medical Care from an Economic Viewpoint*. Santa Monica: Rand Corporation, 1976.

Paddock, William, and Paddock, Paul. *Famine—1975! America's Decision: Who Will Survive?* Boston: Little, Brown and Company, 1967.

The President's Biomedical Research Panel. *The Place of Biomedical Science in Medicine and the State of the Science.* Appendix A of *Report of the President's Biomedical Research Panel.* Washington, D.C.: United States Government Printing Office, 1976.

The Queen v. Dudley and Stephens, 14 Q. B. D. 273 (1884).

Rabinovitch, Nachum L. "Random Mechanisms." *Probability and Statistical Inference in Ancient and Medieval Jewish Literature.* Toronto: University of Toronto Press, 1973.

Shaw, George Bernard. *The Doctor's Dilemma: A Tragedy.* Baltimore: Penguin Books, 1965.

Stone, Deborah A. "Physicians as Gatekeepers: Illness Certification as a Rationing Device." *Public Policy* XXVII (Spring 1979): 227–254.

Turnbull, Colin. *The Mountain People.* New York: Simon and Schuster, 1972.

United States v. Holmes, 26 Fed. Cas. 360 No. 15, 383 (CEED. Pa. 1842).

Weinstein, Milton C., and Stason, William B. "Foundations of Cost-Effectiveness Analysis for Health and Medical Practices." *The New England Journal of Medicine* CCXCVI (March 31, 1977): 716–721.

"Will the U.S. Ration Health Care?" *Perspective* XIV (Winter 1979): 1–5.

Index

223

Designer: Gayle Birrell and Michael Sheridan
Compositor: Freedmen's Organization
Printer: Braun-Brumfield, Inc.
Binder: Braun-Brumfield, Inc.
Text: 10/12 Trump Medieval
Display: 20/24 Trump Medieval

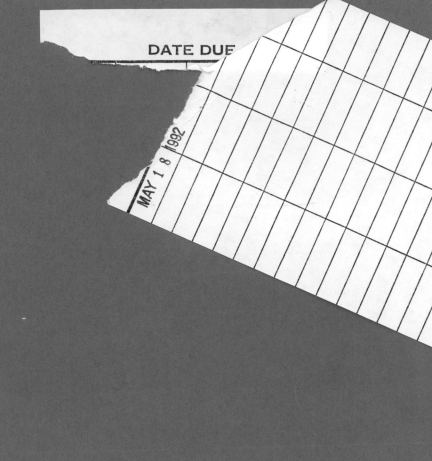

DATE DUE

MAY 1 8 1992

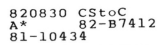